Rheumatology and musculoskeletal disorders

Jessica J. Manson
MBChB MRCP PhD
Consultant Rheumatologist, University College Hospital, London, UK

Sharon A. Chambers
MBBS MRCP MD
Consultant Rheumatologist, Maidstone and Tunbridge Wells NHS Trust, Kent, UK

David A. Isenberg
MD FRCP FAMS
Academic Director and Arthritis Research UK Professor of Rheumatology
Centre for Rheumatology Research, University College London, London, UK

Joan T. Merrill
MD
OMRF Professor of Medicine, University of Oklahoma Health Sciences Center
Head, Clinical Pharmacology Research Program, Oklahoma Medical Research Foundation
Oklahoma City, OK, USA

Michael E. Shipley
MA MD FRCP
Consultant Rheumatologist, University College Hospital, London, UK

CRC Press

CRC Press
Taylor & Francis Group
6000 Broken Sound Parkway NW, Suite 300
Boca Raton, FL 33487-2742

Printed on acid-free paper
Version Date: 20140227

International Standard Book Number-13: 978-1-84076-094-1 (Paperback)

Library of Congress Cataloging-in-Publication Data

Manson, Jessica J., author.
Rapid review of rheumatology and musculoskeletal disorders / Jessica J. Manson, David Isenberg, Sharon Chambers, Michael E. Shipley, Joan T. Merrill.
p. ; cm.
Includes bibliographical references and index.
Summary: "Bringing together a wealth of experience in teaching, research and clinical practice, the authors have produced a concise evidence-based guide to the diagnosis and treatment of rheumatological and related musculoskeletal disorders. The first section, approximately 25% of the book, outlines principles and the necessary clinical skills, ranging from basic science, physical examination and history, to signs, investigations, injection techniques and classification of rheumatological conditions. The central section (approximately 60%) contains 100 case presentations illustrated by clinical color photos and imaging with detailed explanations. Topics covered include autoimmune rheumatic diseases, rheumatoid arthritis, osteoarthritis, bone disease, mechanical disorders, soft tissue, cancer, infections, chronic pain and much more. There is a summary page for each major condition. The interface between primary and hospital care is addressed. The final section deals with data interpretation, such as X-rays, dermatomes and autoantibodies. The rapid review appeals to young doctors/residents in rheumatology and general medicine; primary care physicians, physical therapists and related professionals, senior medical students"--Provided by publisher.
ISBN 978-1-84076-094-1 (paperback : alk paper)
I. Isenberg, David (David Alan), author. II. Chambers, Sharon, 1972- author. III. Shipley, Michael, author. IV. Merrill, Joan T., author. V. Title.
[DNLM; 1. Rheumatic Diseases--diagnosis--Case Reports. 2. Rheumatic Diseases--therapy--Case Reports. 3. Musculoskeletal Diseases--diagnosis--Case Reports. 4. Musculoskeletal Diseases--therapy--Case Reports. WE 544]

RC927
616.7'23--dc23 2014006180

Visit the Taylor & Francis Web site at
http://www.taylorandfrancis.com

and the CRC Press Web site at
http://www.crcpress.com

Contents

Preface

Rheumatology is a joy to practise, and the main purpose of this book is to inspire the reader by providing a taste of what we do. The bulk of the book is made up of cases written by five rheumatologists, with different but overlapping subspecialties and interests. Each case is based on a real patient. The cases cover all kinds of musculoskeletal presentations, from vasculitis to shoulder pain. Some of the cases are short, with an emphasis on spot diagnosis. Some are longer, with more detail in the case and the explanation. This reflects the different kind of involvement you might have with a patient – from spending hours with a particular patient during their stay in hospital, to reviewing them briefly in clinic, to discussing an image or a blood result in a team meeting.

There is a chapter on joint examination, which describes a useful screening musculoskeletal examination, and also more detailed regional examinations to be used when appropriate.

There is a chapter describing our top 10 rheumatological disease categories with links to appropriate cases. There are also two appendices which, respectively, endeavour to demystify the commonly requested autoantibody tests and immunomodulatory drugs which we use.

Our target audience includes doctors and medical students with an interest in rheumatology, or generalists who want to learn more about the specialty, and also nurse specialists, physiotherapists and other allied health professionals.

The key to diagnosis, perhaps in a specialty such as rheumatology in particular, is to think broad and deep. Our patients commonly suffer from multisystem disease, and as such may present in a multitude of ways. Diagnosis is often clinical, and therefore experience and exposure to as many cases as possible is crucial.

As I write this, I am about to go and review a patient with EGPA (Churg–Strauss vasculitis) who presented with a vesicovaginal fistula. You don't see that in many textbooks.

Dr Jessica Manson
Editor

Acknowledgements

Our thanks to Granville Swana, Department of Immunology, Guy's and St. Thomas Hospital, London, for providing the immunofluorescence images for Appendix 1, to Dr Sabrina Valentino, Department of Rheumatology, University College Hospital, London, for help in compiling the normal lab values section and to Mr Fion Bremnar, Department of Ophthalmology, University College Hospital, London, for Figure 2.30.

And finally, to Mike Manson who had the idea for this book and helped bring it to fruition.

Abbreviations

ACA	anti-centromere antibody
ACE	angiotensin converting enzyme
ALP	alkaline phosphatase
ALT	alanine transaminase
ANA	anti-nuclear antibody
ANCA	anti-neutrophil cytoplasmic antibodies
AOSD	adult onset Still's disease
AS	ankylosing spondylitis
ASAS	assessment of spondyloarthritis (classification criteria)
ASO	anti-streptolysin O antibody test
AST	aspartate aminotransferase
ATA	anti-topoisomerase antibodies
AVN	avascular necrosis
BASDAI	Bath ankylosing spondylitis disease activity index
BASFI	Bath ankylosing spondylitis functional index
BCG	bacillus Calmette–Guérin
bd	twice a day
BMD	bone mineral density
BMI	body mass index
BUN	blood urea nitrogen
cANCA	cytoplasmic anti-neutrophil cytoplasmic antibodies
CAPS	catastrophic anti-phospholipid syndrome
CCP	cyclic citrullinated peptide antibody
CH50	complement activity test
CK	creatine kinase
CMC	carpometacarpal (joint)
CMT	Charcot–Marie–Tooth (syndrome)
CNS	central nervous system
CP	chronic periaortitis
Creat	creatinine
CRP	C-reactive protein
CSF	cerebrospinal fluid
CT	computed tomography
CTS	carpal tunnel syndrome
DEXA	dual energy x-ray absorptiometry
DIP	distal interphalangeal (joint)
DISH	diffuse idiopathic skeletal hyperostosis
DM	dermatomyositis
DMARD	disease modifying antirheumatic drugs
dsDNA	double stranded deoxyribonucleic acid
DVT	deep vein thrombosis
ECG	electrocardiogram/electrocardiography
EGPA	eosinophilic granulomatosis with polyangiitis
ELISA	enzyme linked immunosorbent assay
EMG	electromyogram/electromyography
EN	erythema nodosum
ENA	extractable nuclear antigen
ESR	erythrocyte sedimentation rate
FBC	full blood count
FDG	fludeoxyglucose
GALS	gait, arms, legs and spine (locomotor system screen)
GCA	giant cell arteritis
GGT	gamma-glutamyl transpeptidase
GPA	granulomatosis with polyangiitis
Hb	haemoglobin
HbA1c	glycated haemoglobin
HCQ	hydroxychloroquine
HDL	high-density lipoprotein
HELLP	haemolysis/elevated liver enzymes/low platelet count syndrome
HFE	haemochromatosis (gene)
HIV	human immunodeficiency virus
HLA	human leucocyte antigen
IFA	immunofluorescence assay
Ig	immunoglobulin
IL-1	interleukin 1
IL-6	interleukin 6
IM	intramuscular
INR	international normalized ratio
IP	interphalangeal (joint)
ITU	intensive care unit
IV	intravenous

JDM	juvenile dermatomyositis
JIA	juvenile idiopathic arthritis
LDH	lactate dehydrogenase
LE	lupus erythematosus
mAb	monoclonal antibody
MCP	metacarpophalangeal (joint)
MCV	mean cell volume
MPO	myeloperoxidase
MRI	magnetic resonance imaging
MSU	monosodium urate
MTP	metatarsophalangeal
MTX	methotrexate
NCS	nerve conduction studies
NICE	National Institute for Health and Care Excellence
NSAID	non-steroidal anti-inflammatory drug
NTX	N-telopeptide
OA	osteoarthritis
od	once daily
pANCA	perinuclear anti-neutrophil cytoplasmic antibodies
PCR	polymerase chain reaction
PET	positron emission tomography
PIP	proximal interphalangeal (joint)
Plt	platelet
PMR	polymyalgia rheumatica
PO	by mouth
PR3	proteinase 3
PsA	psoriatic arthritis
PSRA	poststreptococcal reactive arthritis
PTH	parathyroid hormone
RA	rheumatoid arthritis
RBC	red blood cell
RDW	red cell distribution width
RF	rheumatoid factor
RNA	ribonucleic acid
RNP	ribonucleoprotein
RP	relapsing polychondritis
RS3PE	remitting seronegative symmetrical synovitis with pitting oedema
S-IBM	sporadic inclusion body myositis
SC	subcutaneous
SD	standard deviation
SLE	systemic lupus erythematosus
SPZ	sulphasalazine
SR	slow release
ssDNA	single stranded deoxyribonucleic acid
TB	tuberculosis
tds	three times a day
TIBC	total iron binding capacity
TNF	tumour necrosis factor
TPMT	thiopurine methyltransferase
TSH	thyroid stimulating hormone test
TTP	thrombotic thrombocytopenic purpura
VAS	visual analogue score
VDRL	Venereal Disease Research Laboratory test
WBC	white blood cells
WHO	World Health Organization

Normal Laboratory Values

ACE	8–52 U/l
albumin	34–50 g/l
ALP	35–104 IU/l
ALT	10–35 IU/l
anti-CCP antibody	0–6.99 units/ml
anti-dsDNA	0–50 IU/ml
anti-cardiolipin antibodies	0–12 GPLU/ml or MPLU/ml
AST	0–37 IU/l (Male) 0–31 IU/l (Female)
B12	191–663 pg/ml
Bence Jones proteins	none detected in normal subjects
bilirubin	0–20 μmol/l
C3	0.90–1.80 g/l
C4	0.10–0.40 g/l
calcium	2.15–2.55 mmol/l
CK	38–204 IU/l (M) 26–140 IU/l (F)
Creat	66–112 μmol/l (M) 48–92 μmol/l (F)
CRP	0.0–5.0 mg/l
cryoglobulins	in normal subjects no cryoproteins are present
ESR	>40 y: 1–20 mm/h <40 y: 1–5 mm/h (M) 1–7 mm/h (F)
ferritin (serum)	13–150 μg/l
folate	4.6–18.7 ng/ml
GGT	10–71 IU/l (M) 6–42 IU/l (F
glucose (serum)	3.9–5.8 mmol/l
Hb	13.0–17.0 g/dl (M) 11.5–15.5 g/dl (F)
HDL	0.9–1.5 mmol/l (M) 1.2–1.7 mmol/l (F)
IgA	0.7–4.0 g/l
IgG	7.0–16.0 g/l
iron	6.6–26.0 μmol/l
LDH	135–225 IU/l (M) 135–214 IU/l (F)
lymphocytes	1.2–3.65 × 10^9/l
magnesium	0.6–1.0 mmol/l
MCV	80–99 fl
neutrophils	2.0–7.5 × 10^9/l
PTH	1.6–6.9 pmol/l
phosphate	0.87–1.45 mmol/l
platelet count	150–400 × 10^9/l
potassium	3.5–5.1 mmol/l
RDW	11.5–15%
reticulocyte count	0.38–2.61%
RF (turbidimetry)	0.0–14.0 IU/ml
sodium	135–145 mmol/l
thyroxine	12.0–22.0 pmol/l
TSH	0.27–4.20 mIU/l
urate	266–474 μmol/l (M) 175–363 μmol/l (F)
urea	1.7–8.3 mmol/l
Urinalysis:	
urine protein	0.0–0.10 g/dl
urine protein:creatinine ratio	0–13.0 mg/mmol
vitamin D	25–120 nmol/l <25 deficient, 25–50 insufficient
WBC	3.0–10.0 × 10^9/l

Chapter 1

MUSCULOSKELETAL EXAMINATION

Many rheumatological conditions do not confine themselves to joints, tendons or muscles. In any patient in whom an inflammatory condition is suspected, a full, general examination should be carried out. In addition, a screening musculoskeletal examination should be part of the assessment of anyone who is unwell.

The required rheumatological examination is dependent upon context. Different knowledge and skills are required to perform a complete assessment of a single symptomatic joint, compared to a broader, screening musculoskeletal examination. The general mantra of 'look, feel, move' holds true for all joints, and this is complemented by a variety of special tests and functional assessments.

Below are a few general points to bear in mind throughout the examination:

- *Is this normal or abnormal?* This sounds very straightforward, but often isn't. The best way to address this problem is to examine as many patients as you can, and get used to the range of normal findings. They differ with age, between the stiff and the hypermobile and with different races.
- *Is there a loss of symmetry?* Asymmetry of joints is almost always an indicator of pathology. The converse is not true, however, and it is important to remember that some illnesses, such as rheumatoid arthritis (RA), classically cause joint disease in a symmetrical distribution (**1.1**).

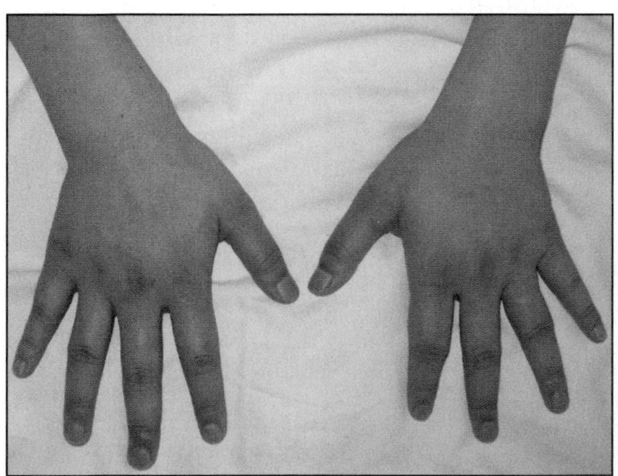

Fig. 1.1 Diffuse, symmetrical swelling of MCP and PIP joints in a 23-year-old woman with early RA.

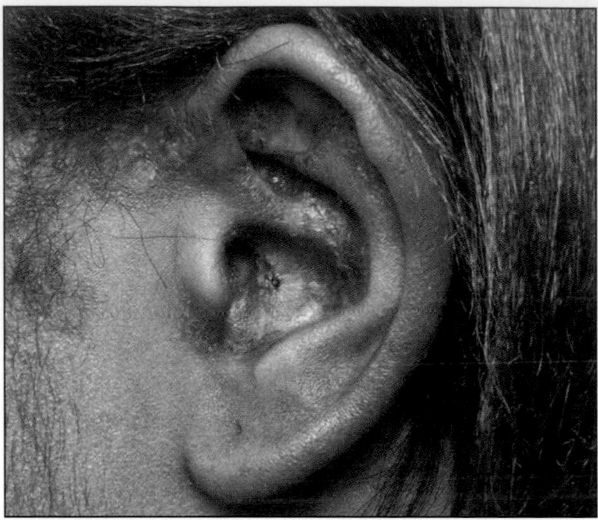

Fig. 1.2 Lesions of discoid lupus in and around the ear of a 19-year-old woman with SLE.

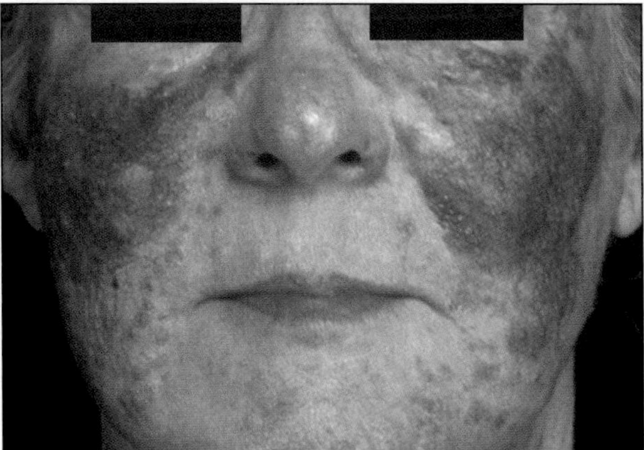

Fig. 1.3 The maculopapular 'butterfly rash' of SLE in a middle-aged woman. (Courtesy of St John's Institute of Dermatology [King's College], Guy's Hospital, London; from: Rycroft et al. [2010] Dermatology, a Colour Handbook, CRC Press.)

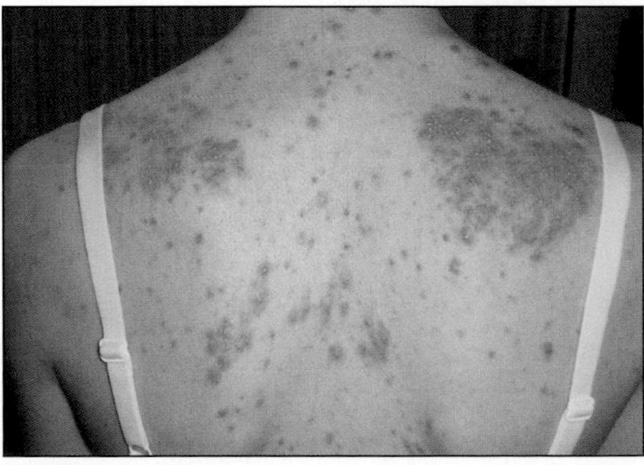

Fig. 1.4 Neutrophilic dermatosis in a 34-year-old woman with adult Sweet's syndrome.

- *Is there a recognizable pattern of disease?* Answering this question requires a basic grasp of the rheumatological diseases, and recognizing these patterns helps you to know how to proceed further with your examination. For instance, RA is often symmetrical and affects the smaller joints whereas spondyloarthropathies usually affect joints asymmetrically. Gout is often a very acute monoarthritis.
- *Is there evidence of a systemic disease?* When starting the examination, ask yourself the important question, 'is this patient sick or well?' This initial inspection gives you the opportunity to glean information about the general health of the patient. In addition, as rheumatological conditions are so often part of a wider, systemic illness, *are there any extra-articular features that may aid the rheumatological diagnosis?* Again, knowing what to look for – for instance the typical rashes of systemic lupus erythematosus (SLE) (**1.2, 1.3**) or rarer rashes such as a neutrophilic dermatosis (**1.4**) – is crucial.
- *Is the patient able to function normally?* As with any examination, assessment of the musculoskeletal system should begin the minute the patient walks into the room. The information available from the patient's gait, the way they get into or out of a chair, and onto the examination couch, provides an immediate insight into the functional impact of any problems they describe.

In addition to the techniques and systems used to assess each specific joint, a screening examination, the GALS (gait, arms, legs, spine) locomotor system screen has been developed. Taking only a few minutes to complete, the GALS screen aims to highlight areas of abnormality, which can then be examined in greater detail if appropriate.

THE GALS LOCOMOTOR SYSTEM SCREEN

It is necessary to have the patient undressed to their underwear.

Gait

Watch the patient walking away from, and back towards you across the room. Ask yourself the following questions:

1 Is the movement smooth and symmetrical?
2 Is there symmetry of the spine?
3 Is the gait normal? Any evidence of an antalgic (limping) gait – protection of one limb because of pain?

Ask the patient to get onto the examination couch.

Arms

Carry out a general inspection of the skin and muscle bulk with the patient sitting. Then, start by looking at the hands. Flexing the elbows, and keeping the arms adducted, ask the patient to show you the palmar and then the dorsal aspects of their hands; watch the way they move – this provides clues as to areas of pathology. Look for swelling, deformity or redness of the joints. It is also useful to assess the nails, looking in particular for evidence of psoriasis (**1.5**) or abnormal nail fold capillaries (**1.6**). Ask the patient to make a fist, at which point you can assess their grip, and to make a pincer between the thumb and each finger on one hand, and then the other. These are both functionally very important movements. Some people advocate the metacarpal squeeze, though judge carefully on whom to perform this test – it can be very uncomfortable, and unnecessary, in the context of gross synovitis of the metacarpophalangeal (MCP) joints. Can the patient fully extend both elbows, or is one restricted? Can they pronate and supinate the hand? Can they get their palms and fingers flat together with their wrists at 90° of dorsal and palmar flexion?

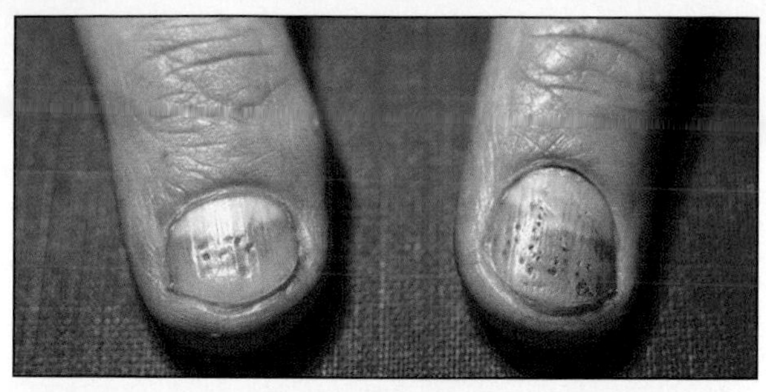

a

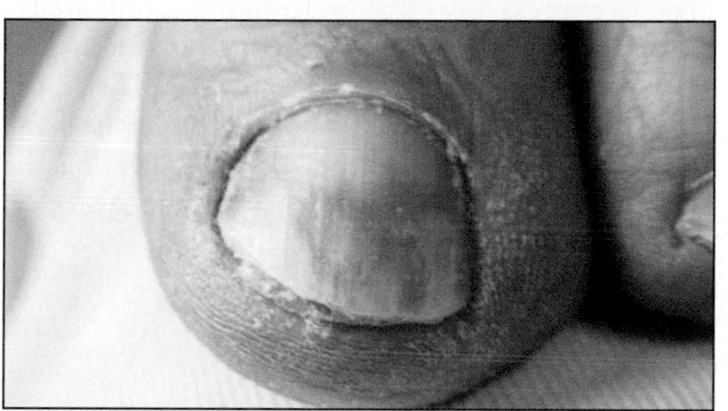

b

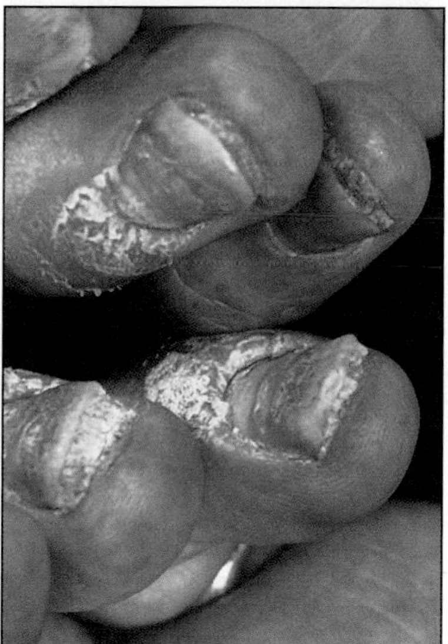

c

Fig. 1.5 Nail changes of psoriasis: pitting (**1.5a**), onycholysis (**1.5b**), subungual hyperkeratosis (**1.5c**). (Courtesy of Menter & Stoff [2010] Psoriasis, CRC Press.)

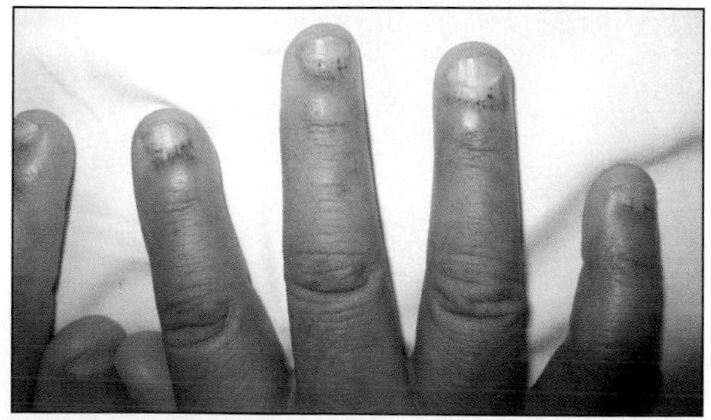

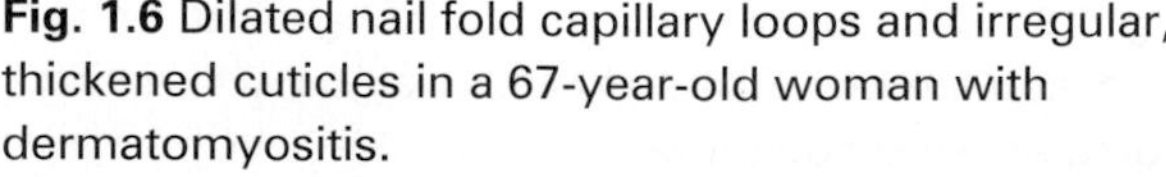

Fig. 1.6 Dilated nail fold capillary loops and irregular, thickened cuticles in a 67-year-old woman with dermatomyositis.

Next, ask the patient to put both their hands behind their head and back. This is pretty much impossible in the presence of significant shoulder or elbow pathology.

Legs

With the patient lying on the couch, first inspect the knees for swelling, redness or deformity. Assess for an effusion (**1.7**) by two methods. The patellar tap test is performed by cupping the thigh just above the knee to express any effusion from the suprapatellar pouch and maximize the fluid content of the knee. Then gently press down on the patella. The test is positive when the patella is felt to bounce back up to your fingers after a slight delay, indicating the presence of a large effusion. You may also feel fluctuance in the suprapatellar pouch.

The 'bulge test' is better for detecting small amounts of fluid. Cup the thigh again, and then sweep the medial aspect of the joint from top to bottom. Keeping your eye on this area, sweep the outer aspect. Fluid in the knee will then appear as a slow bulging on the medial aspect of the knee.

Flex each knee and hip in turn while feeling across the top of the knee for crepitus. Also check hip internal rotation.

Look at the feet for deformities (**1.8**), and the soles for callosities, then check for joint tenderness with the metatarsal squeeze test, remembering that it may cause pain.

Spine

This part of the examination should ideally be done after the gait assessment. Look at the patient standing from behind and both sides looking for any abnormal curvature of the spine – exaggerated kyphosis or lordosis, or scoliosis. The 'four point test' is a quick and easy way of assessing spinal alignment. Ask the patient to stand against a wall; with a normal spine, there should be four points of contact: the heels, buttocks, shoulder blades and occiput, with a normal lumbar lordosis.

Next, ask the patient to bend forward and attempt to touch their toes, while keeping their knees extended. Normal flexion should be sufficient to separate fingers placed on adjacent lumbar vertebrae (the modified Schober's test). Check the spinous processes for bony tenderness (rare) or pain on percussion and the paraspinal muscles for tender muscle spasm (much more common). Similarly, assess cervical spine movements with lateral flexion of the neck, a sensitive test for pathology in this area.

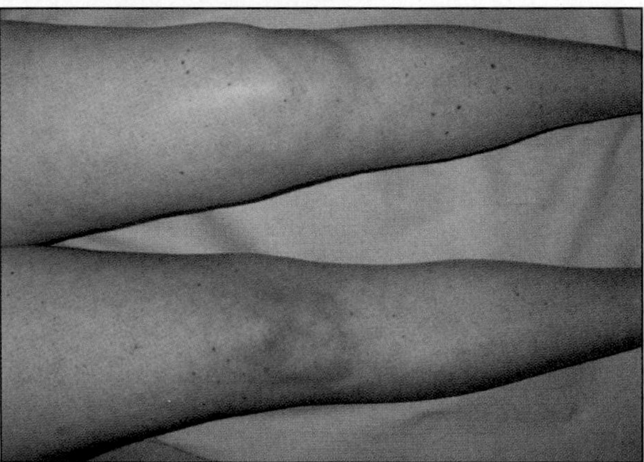

Fig. 1.7 An effusion affecting the left knee of a 20-year-old woman with RA.

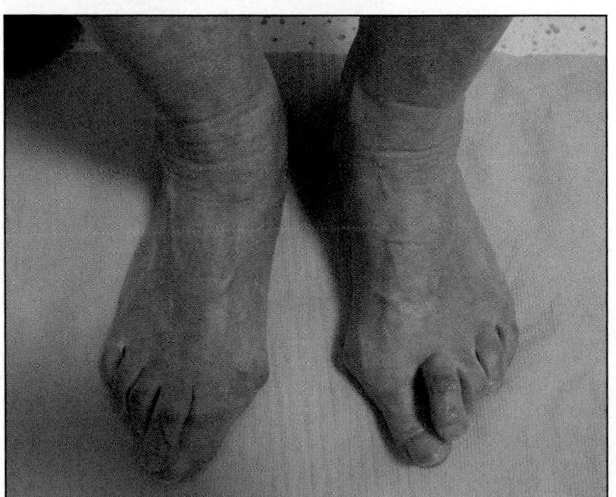

Fig. 1.8 A 73-year-old woman with longstanding RA involving the feet. Bilateral hallux valgus with over-riding of the second toes.

REGIONAL EXAMINATION

The hands

In addition to 'look, feel, move', it is useful to think 'nail, skin, muscles, joints' when looking at the hands. It is a good start to ask the patient to expose their arms to above the elbows. This may reveal either rheumatoid nodules (**1.9**) or plaque psoriasis (**1.10**), and is also an early hint of the patient's functional status. As mentioned above, examine the nails for signs of psoriasis (pitting, onycholysis, subungual hyperkeratosis, yellow-brown discolouration), systemic sclerosis and dermatomyositis (nail bed capillary dilatation and cuticle cragginess; see **1.6**) and vasculitis (nail fold infarcts, splinter haemorrhages). Systemic sclerosis is also associated with calcinosis (**1.11**) in the finger tip pulp. This needs to be differentiated from the urate deposits seen in tophaceous gout (**1.12**).

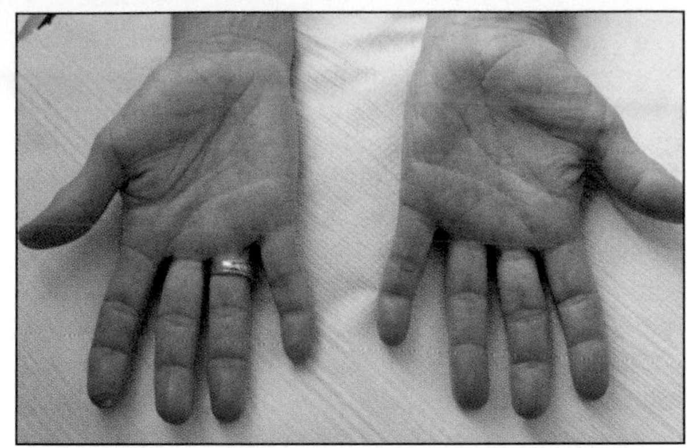

Fig. 1.11 Calcinosis affecting the tip of the right index finger in a 52-year-old woman with limited cutaneous systemic sclerosis.

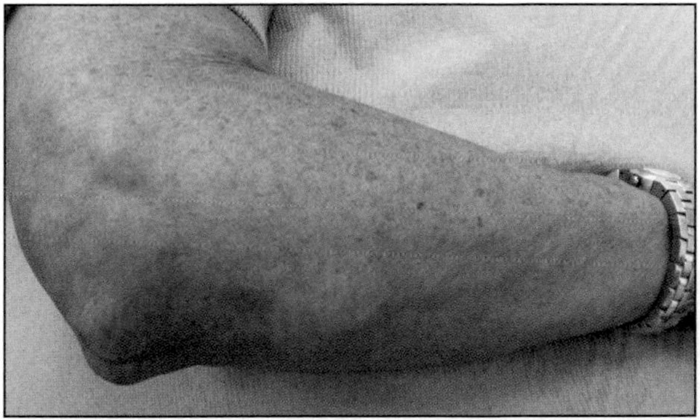

Fig. 1.9 Rheumatoid nodules over the extensor surface of the elbow of a 58-year-old woman with seropositive RA. Note that the more proximal nodule returned after surgery, a common problem.

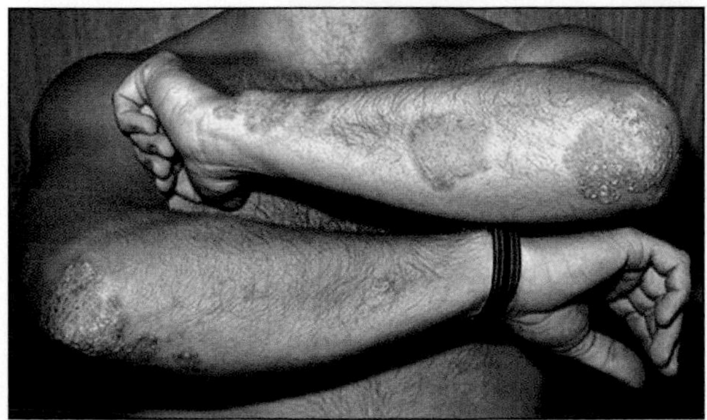

Fig. 1.10 Plaque psoriasis over the elbows. (Courtesy of Menter & Stoff [2010] *Psoriasis*, CRC Press.)

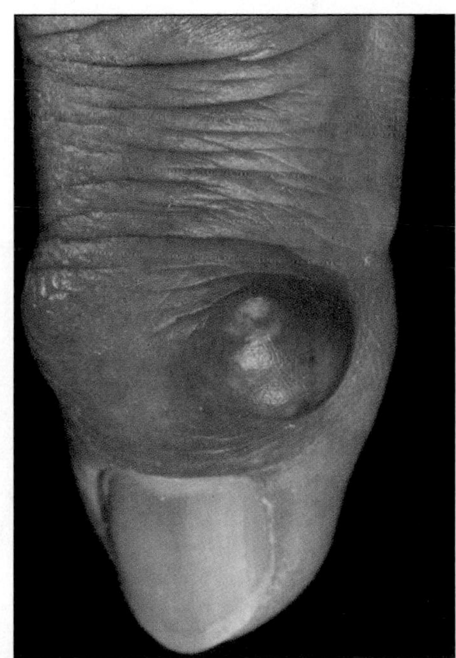

Fig. 1.12 A gouty tophus overlying the PIP joint of the right index finger of a 70-year-old man with chronic tophaceous gout.

The skin of the hands and arms may be affected by psoriasis, or show further evidence of vasculitis, either secondary to RA, or as part of a primary vasculitis. Discoid lupus (**1.13**) can affect the hands. Tightness of the skin and distal spindling of the fingers is a feature of systemic sclerosis (**1.14**). The skin may also provide insights into previous therapy – for instance the thinning and easy bruising seen with long-term corticosteroid use (**1.15**).

As can also be seen in **Figure 1.15**, loss of general muscle bulk may be indicative of disuse, secondary to pain from arthritis, or due to drugs, particularly corticosteroids. More specifically, wasting of the thenar eminence results from median nerve compression, or carpal tunnel syndrome, which is a complication of arthritis affecting the wrist and of flexor tenosynovitis, and can be a complication of inflammatory arthritis.

Inspect the joints, starting at the wrist and moving distally. Look for swelling, redness and deformity. Compare with the other side. Palpate the joint, first for warmth, indicating active inflammation, and then for swelling. Swelling can be bony, either from osteoarthritic change or from 'burnt out' arthritis with secondary damage, or 'boggy', due to ongoing synovitis. Some swelling can be due to disease in the overlying tendon sheath (**1.16**, in this case due to overuse). Be careful when squeezing an actively inflamed joint. It can be very painful. Blanching of your nail is a good guide as to the degree of pressure to apply. Rheumatoid arthritis classically affects the wrist, MCP and proximal interphalangeal (PIP) joints and is symmetrical. In the longer term it can cause some characteristic deformities – swan neck (reversible or fixed hyperextension at the PIP and flexion at the distal interphalangeal [DIP] joint), boutonnière (flexion at the PIP and hyperextension at the DIP) (**1.17**) and subluxation or ulnar drift at the MCPs (**1.18**).

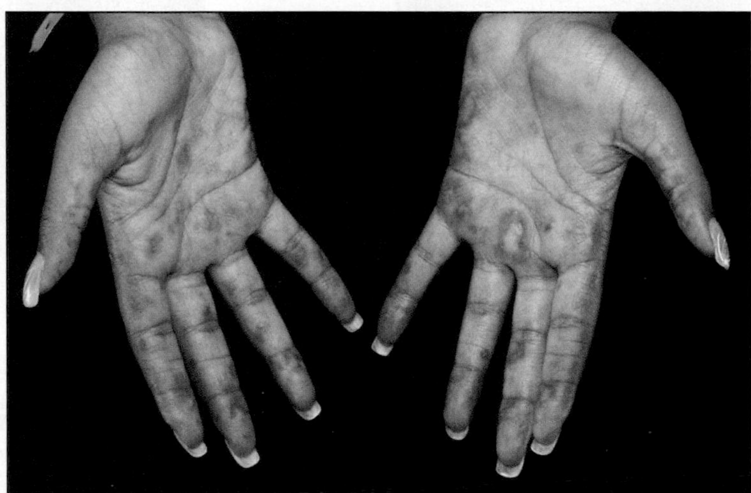

Fig. 1.13 Healing discoid lupus on the hands of a 19-year-old woman with SLE.

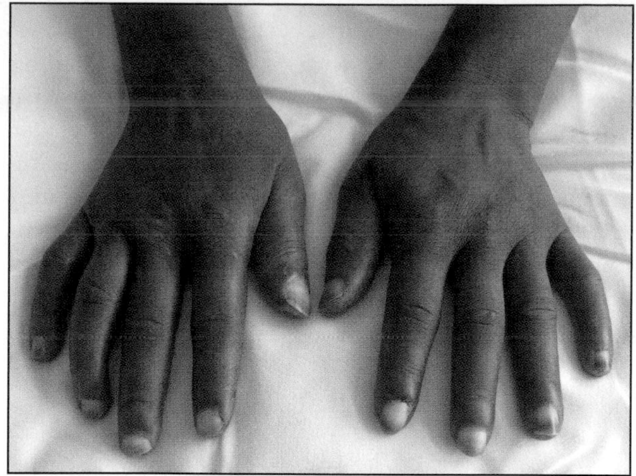

Fig. 1.14 Tightness of skin (sclerodactyly) distally affecting the hands of a 34-year-old woman with limited cutaneous systemic sclerosis. Note also the evidence of digital infarcts.

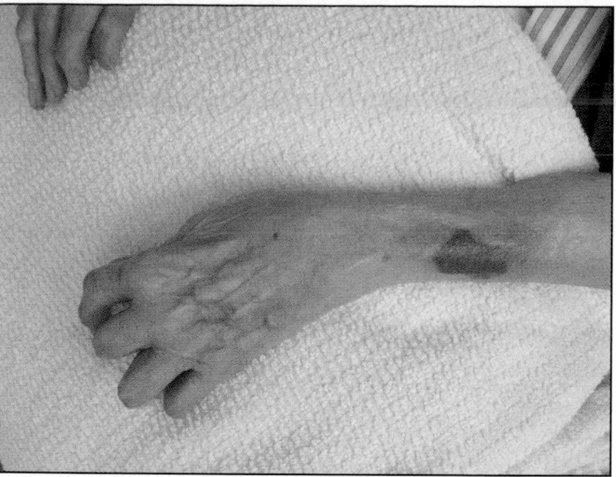

Fig. 1.15 Thinning of the skin, easy bruising and muscle wasting in a 78-year-old woman with long-standing RA treated with corticosteroids.

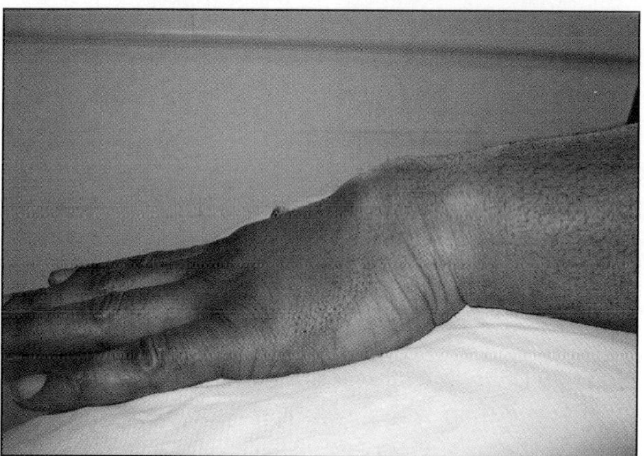

Fig. 1.16 Swelling over the dorsum of the wrist due to a mechanical tenosynovitis of the extensor tendon sheath in a 43-year-old man who was a martial arts enthusiast.

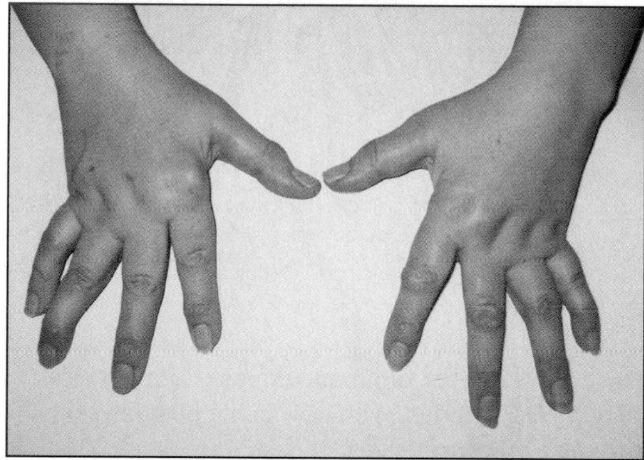

Fig. 1.17 Swan neck deformities of the right ring finger and left little finger, and boutonnière deformity of the left ring finger in a 46-year-old woman with RA.

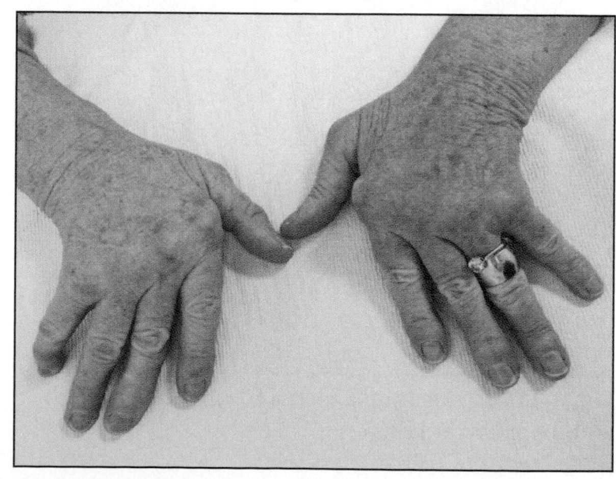

Fig. 1.18 Long-standing RA in a 73-year-old woman, showing ulnar drift and subluxation of the MCP joints.

By contrast, although psoriatic arthritis (PsA) can cause a rheumatoid-like pattern, it can also involve the DIPs and nails (**1.19**), just one or two joints at a time, or sometimes a whole finger or toe (dactylitis or 'sausage digit') (**1.20**). Rarely, it causes a very destructive form of polyarthritis called arthritis mutilans (**1.21**). Osteoarthritis usually manifests in the hands as Heberden's nodes on the DIPs or Bouchard's nodes on the PIPs (**1.22**). It can also cause squaring of the hand as a result of stiffness and adduction of the first carpometacarpal (CMC) joint.

Jaccoud's arthropathy (**1.23**) is seen most commonly in patients with SLE. It is a deforming but non-erosive condition, caused by disease affecting the tendons.

To test movements, start at the wrist, assessing extension and flexion by making the 'prayer' and 'inverse prayer' signs. Movements of the small joints of the hand should be assessed by checking grip and pincer, as described above.

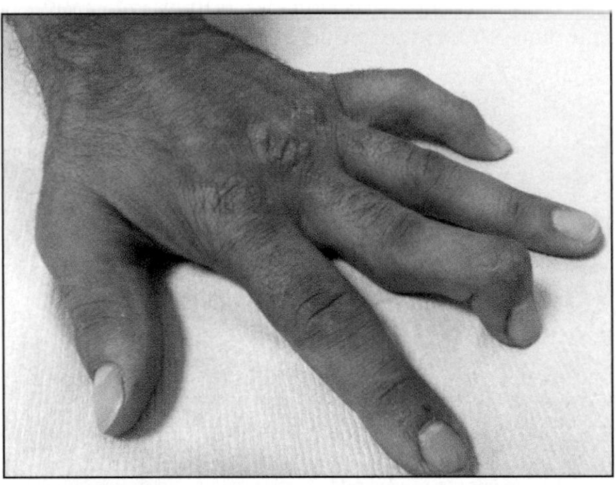

Fig. 1.19 A 33-year-old man with psoriatic arthritis causing DIP arthritis, with noticeable plaques of psoriasis on his knuckles.

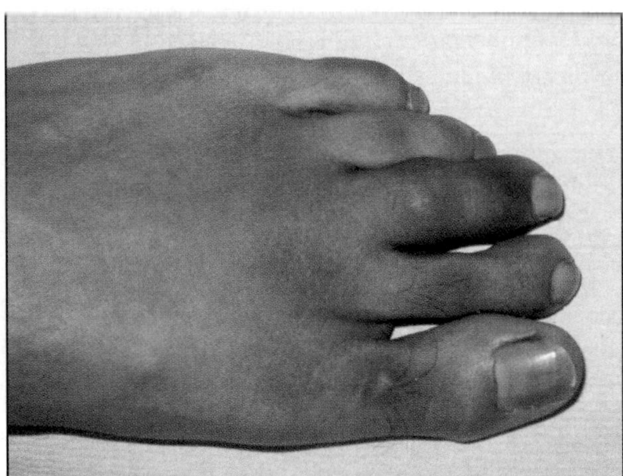

Fig. 1.20 Dactylitis affecting the middle toe in a 30-year-old man with new onset psoriatic arthritis.

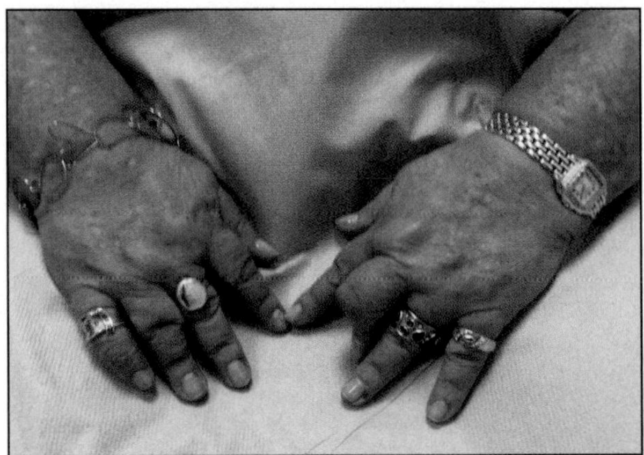

Fig. 1.21 Arthritis mutilans in a 57-year-old woman with psoriatic arthritis.

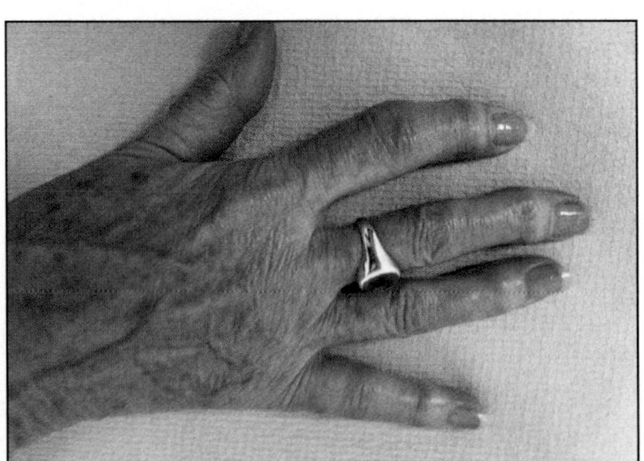

Fig. 1.22 Heberden's (DIP) and Bouchard's (PIP) nodes in a 75-year-old woman with osteoarthritis.

The elbows

Any significant pathology, such as that seen with synovitis (or rarely osteoarthritis), of the elbow joint prevents full extension (**1.24**). More common conditions such as tennis and golfer's elbow cause pain around the elbow, due to an enthesitis affecting the lateral and medial epicondyles respectively. In this case, movements of the elbow will be full, unless restricted by pain. Olecranon bursitis (**1.25**) can be mechanical, part of an inflammatory arthritis, or due to infection or crystal arthropathy.

The shoulder

The shoulder is a very complex structure, and a multitude of eponymous test and signs have been developed to aid clinical diagnosis. The important thing is to differentiate between the main types of pathology. First, do the symptoms (usually pain and restricted movement) originate from the shoulder itself, or from the neck and shoulder girdle? Usually, but not always, this can be determined by testing whether neck or shoulder movements precipitate pain. Ask the patient to show you precisely where

a

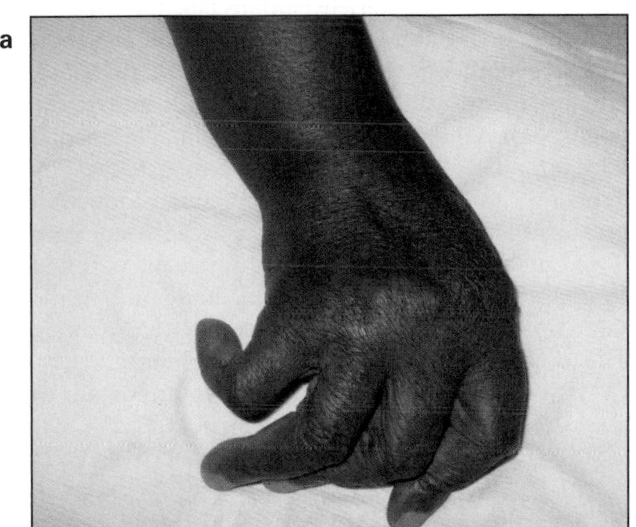

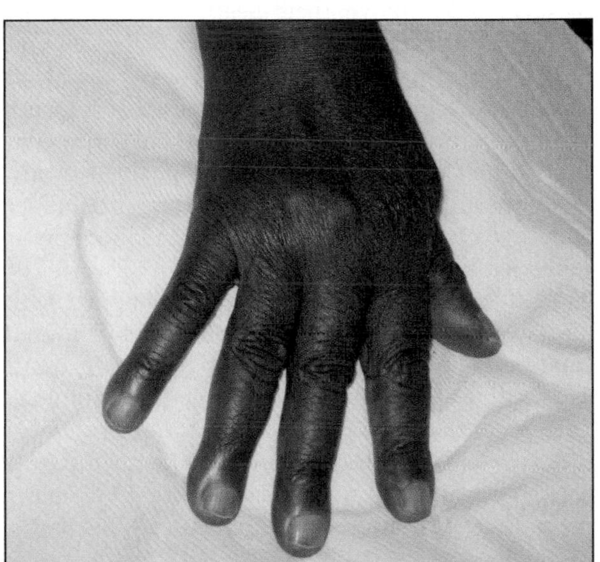

b

Fig. 1.23 Jaccoud's arthropathy at rest (**1.23a**) and when fingers fully extended (**1.23b**) showing that changes are not fixed.

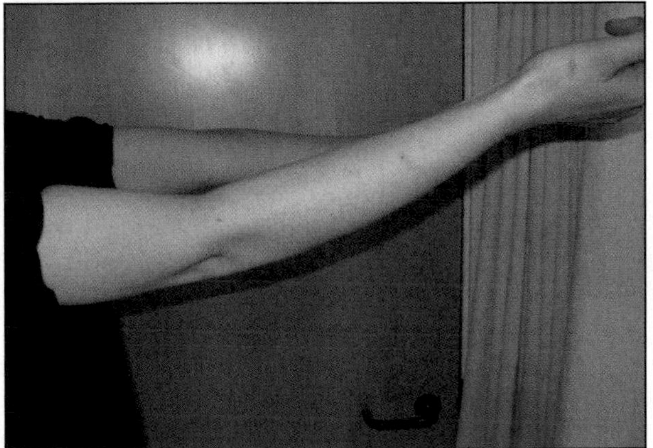

Fig. 1.24 Fixed flexion deformity of the right elbow in a patient with oligoarticular juvenile idiopathic arthritis.

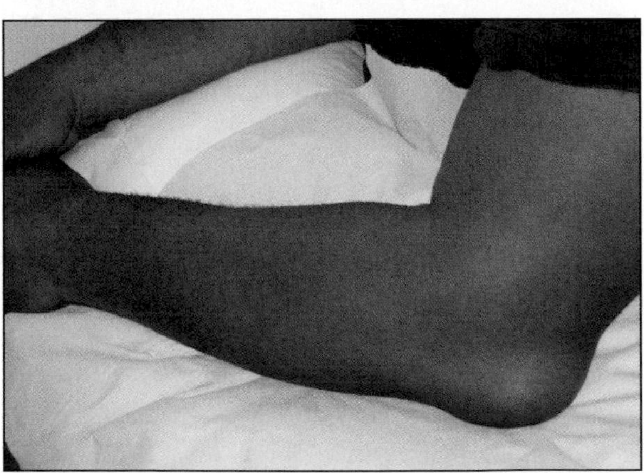

Fig. 1.25 Mechanical olecranon bursitis.

the pain is. True shoulder pain arising from the joint or the rotator cuff is often felt over the deltoid and into the upper arm, whereas pain from cervical spondylosis and paraspinal muscle spasm is felt predominantly at the base of the neck and into the trapezius muscles (shoulder girdle pattern pain). Pathology in the acromioclavicular joint is often well localized to the site of that joint.

Start your examination with the patient standing, facing away from you. Look for asymmetry due to muscle wasting or winging of the scapulae. Assess posture, and the angle at which the patient holds their head. Ask them to turn to face you, and then with arms straight, and palms facing forward, ask them to abduct their arms in an arc, aiming for them to meet above their head. This should be an easy, symmetrical, pain-free movement. If not, this suggests pathology in the glenohumeral or acromioclavicular joints, or affecting the soft tissues of the rotator cuff. A complete lack of movement (so bad that the patient is typically unable to wash under the affected arm!) is seen in a frozen shoulder (adhesive capsulitis). Rotator cuff tendonopathy is suggested by a painful arc (classically between 70° and 120° of abduction) with a positive impingement test (such as abduction to 90° followed by internal rotation in supraspinatus pathology). Rotator cuff tears will result in incomplete abduction. Pathology affecting the acromioclavicular joint often results in localized tenderness, and there are a number of tests which stress the joint, such as adducting by pulling the outstretched arm behind the patient's back.

The knee

A basic examination of the knee is described in the section above on the GALS screen. As with the arms, look for rashes that may help with a rheumatological diagnosis (**1.26**). In addition, there are a number of tests that are used to assess the stability of the knee. Lack of stability, which produces the symptom of the knee 'giving way', is classically associated with ligamentous laxity or tears. Importantly, however, giving way is most commonly due to weak quadriceps, a frequent complication of osteoarthritis or any painful condition of the knee. The anterior and posterior cruciate ligaments prevent slide of the tibia on the femur, anteriorly and posteriorly respectively. To test them, with the patient supine flex the knee to 90°, then anchor the femur by sitting on the foot. Clasping both hands around the top of the tibia, attempt to draw it forwards and back across the femur. Normal slip is less than 0.5 cm. The medial and lateral collateral ligaments are stressed by applying contrasting abduction and adduction pressures above and below the knee, with the knee flexed at about 20°. The medial ligament is tested by abducting at the ankle with one hand, and at the same time pushing the knee medially with the other. This is reversed to test the lateral ligament.

With the patient standing, it is also important to assess for any valgus or varus deformity (**1.27**).

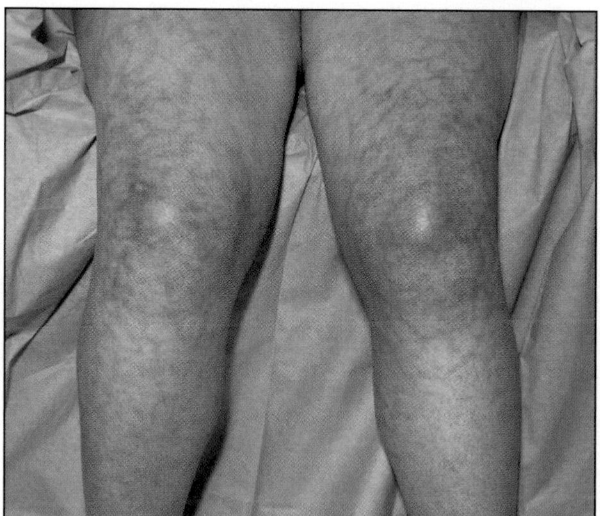

Fig. 1.26 Florid livedo reticularis is a patient with SLE and anti-phospholipid syndrome.

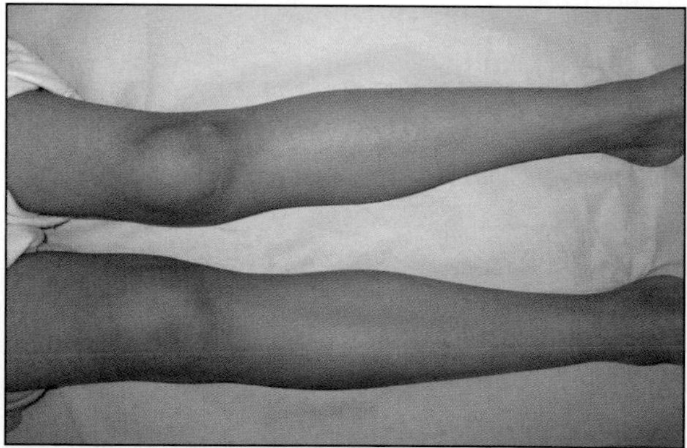

Fig. 1.27 Valgus deformity and effusion of the left knee in a 19-year-old with polyarticular juvenile idiopathic arthritis.

The hip

'Hip' pain very often doesn't actually arise from the hip itself. It is therefore very important to examine more widely when attempting to account for a patient's symptoms. Pain in the buttock may well arise from the sacroiliac joint or the lumbar spine. Tenderness around the hip/buttock is usually due to a bursitis or tendonitis. For instance, trochanteric bursitis, which produces lateral thigh/hip pain, can be diagnosed by finding a tender point on palpation of the greater trochanter of the femur.

With the patient lying supine, flex the hip as far as is comfortable with the knee in flexion (should be about 120°). With the knee flexed to 90°, internally and externally rotate the hip. Normal is about 30° for internal rotation, and 45° for external rotation. Internal rotation is often the first movement to be restricted or painful in the presence of hip pathology. Abduction and adduction are assessed with the knee extended, and extension requires the patient to be lying prone.

The foot and ankle

A useful tip when investigating symptoms in the foot or ankle is to look at the patient's shoe; abnormal wear pattern may help with the diagnosis, and lead you to refer to a podiatrist for suitable orthotics. With the patient standing, check the medial longitudinal arches (**1.28**), then ask the patient to lie on the couch. As mentioned above, look at the sole of the foot for callosities. Check for tenderness at the insertion of the plantar fascia in patients with heel pain, and palpate for localized tenderness in patients with forefoot pain. Assess movements of the ankle – flexion and extension, inversion and eversion – and for any tenderness along the joint line.

The spine

The GALS screen examination of the spine is adequate for many patients. The sciatic nerve stretch test is carried on with the patient supine on the couch. Keeping the knee extended, passively flex the hip by lifting the ankle. Ask the patient to inform when the test becomes uncomfortable. At this limit, passively flex the ankle. A positive test, indicating irritation of the sciatic nerve, produces paraesthesia, numbness or pain below the knee. The most common finding is a pulling sensation in the hamstrings which is not indicative of sciatic nerve pathology. The femoral stretch test is carried out with the patient lying prone. If the test is positive, passive extension of the hip produces spasm in the hamstring and sensory symptoms in the anterior thigh. It is almost always appropriate to carry out a full neurological examination of the upper and lower limbs in a patient who complains of neck or back pain.

Finally, Schober's test is used to assess flexibility of the lumbosacral spine. It is reduced in patients with spondyloarthropathy, such as ankylosing spondylitis, and can be used to assess the progression of their disease.

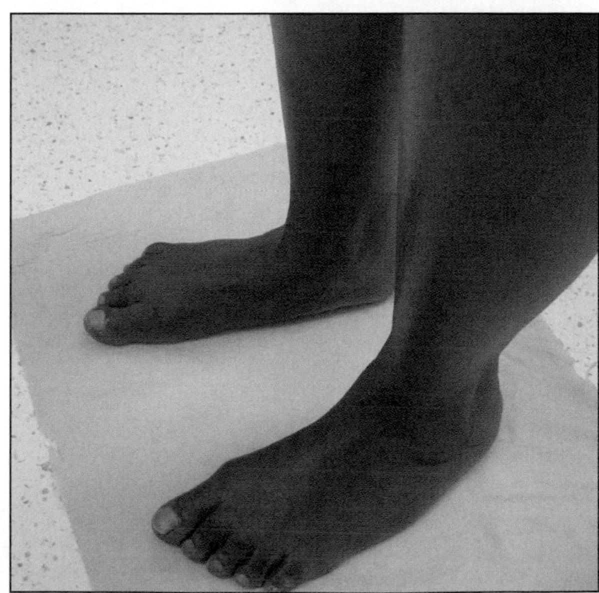

Fig. 1.28 Loss of the medial longitudinal arch, with over-pronation of the ankle and an early hallux valgus on the left foot in a 45-year-old woman with bilateral foot and ankle pain.

Chapter 2

TOP 10 RHEUMATOLOGICAL DISEASE CATEGORIES

The bulk of a general rheumatologist's workload will be the management of patients with inflammatory arthritis and the autoimmune rheumatic diseases such as lupus. In primary care, however, the majority of musculoskeletal symptoms will be non-inflammatory in origin. This list of the top 10 rheumatological disease categories is intended to include a combination of inflammatory and non-inflammatory conditions. Additional conditions are included in the cases.

1 Rheumatoid arthritis
2 Seronegative spondyloarthropathies
3 Systemic lupus erythematosus and the autoimmune rheumatic diseases
4 Crystal arthropathies
5 Vasculitides, including giant cell arteritis and polymyalgia rheumatica
6 Osteoarthritis
7 Chronic widespread pain/fibromyalgia
8 Back pain and other regional soft tissue disorders
9 Osteoporosis and metabolic bone disease
10 Miscellaneous rheumatological conditions

1 RHEUMATOID ARTHRITIS

See cases 11, 25, 26, 28, 34, 38, 73, 85, 86

Definition and clinical features

Rheumatoid arthritis (RA) is the prototypical inflammatory arthritis, which causes a symmetrical destructive polyarthritis and usually involves the small joints of the hands and/or feet. Patients complain of significant early morning stiffness (longer than 30 minutes) with other systemic features such as fatigue.

Patients can experience a wide variety of extra-articular features (see *Table 2.1, overleaf*).

Epidemiology

The prevalence of RA is about 1% in Caucasian populations, but much lower (0.1%) in some rural African populations. Female:male ratio is approximately 3:1. Risk factors are both genetic (HLA-DRB1) and environmental (smoking).

Differential diagnosis

- Seronegative spondyloarthropathies – tend to involve the spine and lower limbs, typically rheumatoid factor (RF) negative, associated with psoriasis and inflammatory bowel disease
- Systemic lupus erythematosus (SLE) – positive anti-nuclear antibody (ANA), numerous systemic features, typically non-deforming arthritis (Jaccoud's arthropathy) if RF negative, generally thrombocytopenia rather than thrombocytosis
- Viral arthritis – usually short lived
- Osteoarthritis – a different pattern of joint involvement, commonly involves distal interphalangeal (DIP) joints, no systemic features, normal inflammatory markers
- Gout – often monoarticular or asymmetrical, raised uric acid, tophi, rapid onset flares.

Investigations

Tests should be performed for raised inflammatory markers (although, importantly, not always present), anaemia of chronic disease and thrombocytosis (*Table 2.2*). Positive RF is seen in approximately 70% of patients (RF positivity confers a relatively poor prognosis); anti-cyclic citrullinated peptide (anti-CCP) has a similar sensitivity to RF, but a much higher specificity (95%). In both cases, higher titres are associated with improved specificity. Radiology includes plain films, ultrasound and magnetic resonance imaging (MRI).

Table 2.1 Extra-articular features of rheumatoid arthritis

Constitutional	Fatigue, malaise, anorexia
Skin	Rheumatoid nodules, cutaneous vasculitis, leg ulcers
Pulmonary	Interstitial fibrosis, pleuritis, pleural effusion (typically exudates), pulmonary rheumatoid nodules, Caplan's syndrome, bronchiolitis obliterans, organizing pneumonia
Cardiac	Poricarditis, pericardial effusion
Haematological	Anaemia of chronic disease, eosinophilia, Felty's syndrome (neutropenia and splenomegaly), large granular lymphocyte syndrome
Gastrointestinal	Elevated liver enzymes (especially alkaline phosphatase)
Neurological	Entrapment neuropathies, e.g. carpal tunnel syndrome, cord compression (cervical disease)
Renal	Amyloidosis, interstitial nephritis
Ocular	Keratoconjunctivitis sicca, episcleritis, scleritis

Table 2.2 The 2010 American College of Rheumatology/European League Against Rheumatism classification criteria for rheumatoid arthritis

Target population (who should be tested?):

Patients who:

1. Have at least one joint with definite clinical synovitis (swelling)
2. With the synovitis not better explained by another disease

Classification criteria for RA (score based algorithm: add score of categories (A–D); a score of ≥6/10 is needed for classification of a patient having definite RA)

A. Joint involvement	
1 large joint	0
2–10 large joints	1
1–3 small joints (with or without involvement of large joints)	2
4–10 small joints (with or without involvement of large joints)	3
>10 joints (at least 1 small joint)	5
B. Serology	
Negative RF and negative anti-CCP	0
Low-positive RF or low-positive anti-CCP	2
High-positive RF or high-positive anti-CCP	3
C. Acute phase reactants	
Normal CRP and normal ESR	0
Abnormal CRP or abnormal ESR	1
D. Duration of symptoms	
<6 weeks	0
≥6 weeks	1

Adapted from Aletaha *et al.* (2010).

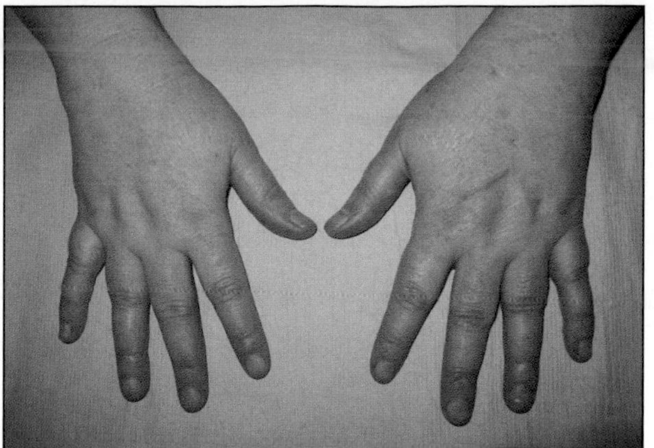

Fig. 2.1 A 43-year-old woman with early RA. This photograph shows non-specific puffiness particularly around the MCPs, with loss of guttering.

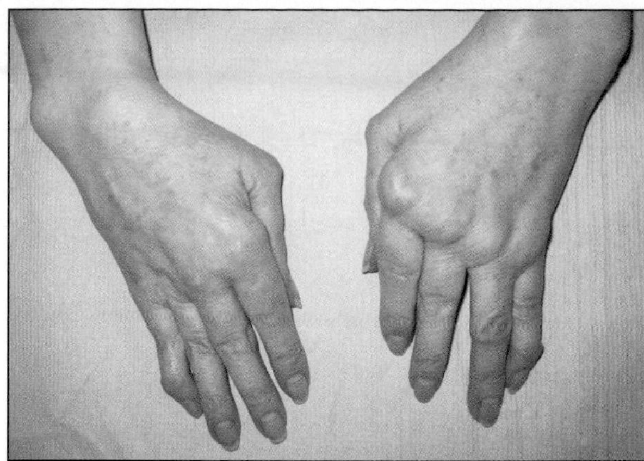

Fig. 2.2 A 62-year-old woman with long-standing RA showing fixed deformities at the wrists, subluxation of the MCPs and swan necking, particularly of the right little finger.

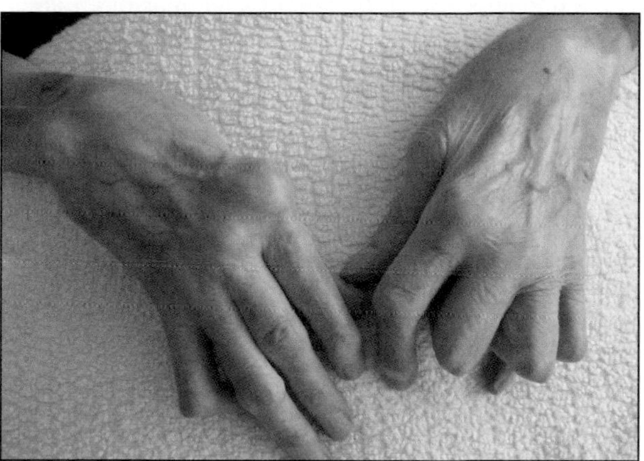

Fig. 2.3 A 79-year-old woman with advanced RA changes. In addition to non-reducible deformities of the joints there is significant loss of muscle bulk and thinning and easy bruising of the skin from steroid use.

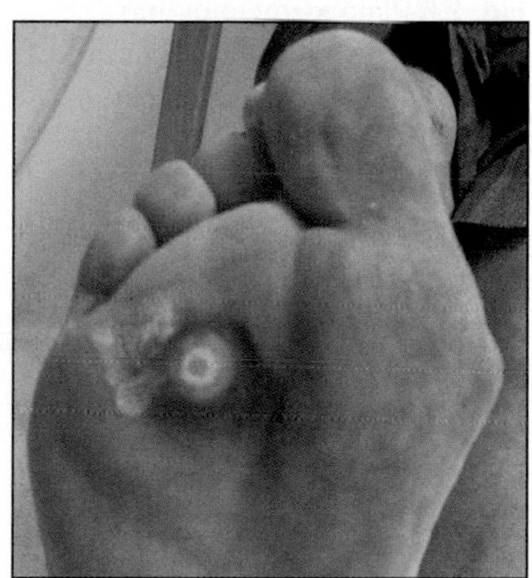

Fig. 2.4 Hallux valgus and corn formation over metatarsal dislocation in a 70-year-old woman with RA.

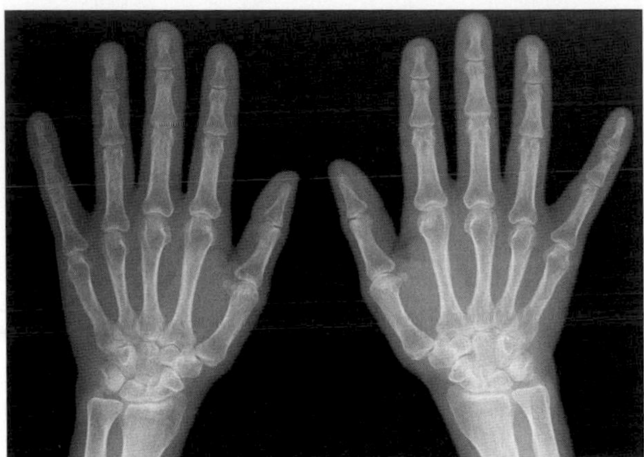

Fig. 2.5 Plain x-ray showing changes of early RA – periarticular osteopenia with reduced joint space particularly around the MCPs.

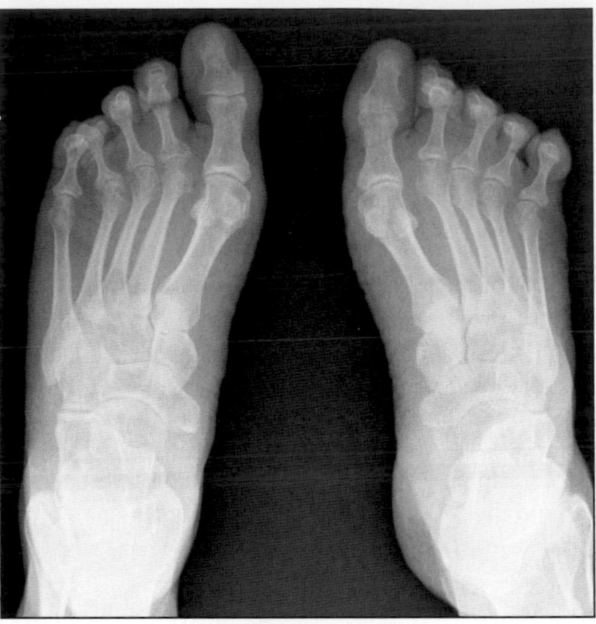

Fig. 2.6 Plain x-ray of the feet of a 64-year-old man with established RA showing periarticular osteopenia of the MTP joints, worse on the left than the right, and joint erosions particularly affecting the left second MTP.

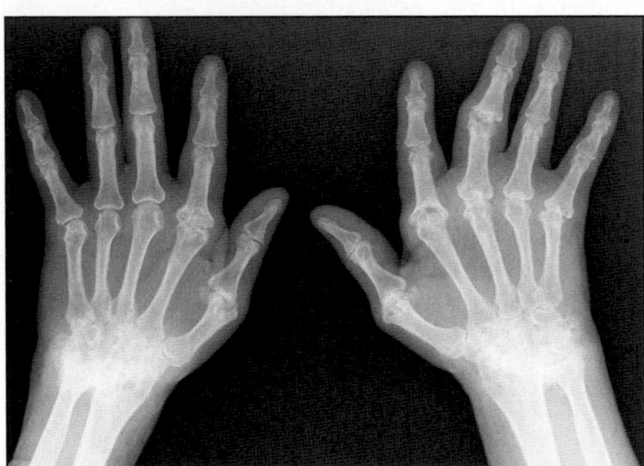

Fig. 2.7 Plain x-ray of hands in long-standing destructive RA – generalized osteopenia, fusion of both wrists with obliteration of joint spaces, erosive changes at MCPs and PIPs with destruction of the metacarpal heads and associated subluxation of the MCPs.

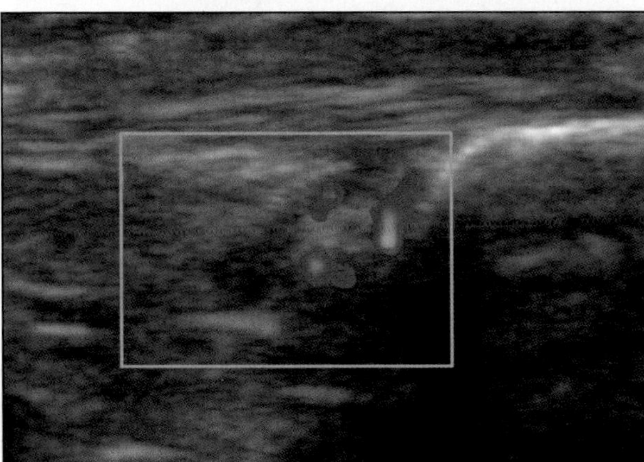

Fig. 2.8 Ultrasound of a 24-year-old man with mildly swollen wrists, confirming significant synovial hypertrophy and increased Doppler signal consistent with active synovitis.

2 SERONEGATIVE SPONDYLOARTHROPATHIES

See cases 5, 50, 64, 82, 89, 100

Definition and clinical features

This group of inflammatory arthritides includes ankylosing spondylitis (AS), psoriatic arthritis (PsA), reactive arthritis, inflammatory bowel disease-associated arthritis and the conditions known as the undifferentiated spondyloarthropathies, which can have features of each of the preceding diagnoses. Typically a patient with a spondyloarthropathy will have inflammatory back pain (worse during the night or in the early morning, better with exercise, associated with significant stiffness) and/or an asymmetric, often predominantly lower limb, peripheral joint arthritis. Other musculoskeletal features include sacroiliitis, which causes buttock pain, enthesopathy and dactylitis. Articular features, particularly involving the axial skeleton, typically respond well to non-steroidal anti-inflammatory drugs (NSAIDs). Extra-articular features which may help to distinguish between the diagnoses are inflammatory bowel disease, psoriasis and urethritis. There is also an association with uveitis.

Epidemiology

Prevalence varies between different populations, but on average, AS affects about 1% of the population. Unlike RA, the spondyloarthropathies are more common in men than in women. The association with the MHC-I antigen HLA-B27 means that spondyloarthropathies often cluster in families. Infective triggers (e.g. *Chlamydia*, *Campylobacter* spp.) have clearly been identified in reactive arthritis.

Differential diagnosis

In patients with a history of antecedent infection, where the diagnosis of reactive arthritis is being considered, it is clearly important to exclude ongoing infections prior to consideration of the use of steroids.

PsA can look clinically similar to RA or AS, or it can take on more distinct patterns – distal interphalangeal (DIP) arthritis associated with psoriatic nail disease and the very severe, and now very rare, arthritis mutilans.

Investigations

The seronegativity relates to having a negative RF. About 90% of patients with AS are HLA-B27 positive, however HLA-B27 positivity of up to 50% can be seen in the unaffected population, limiting its usefulness as a diagnostic tool. Patients with a spondyloarthropathy can have elevated inflammatory markers, but often do not.

The presence of sacroiliitis is central to the diagnosis of AS, and changes can be seen on plain x-ray. MRI is more sensitive, allowing the detection of sacroiliac joint changes earlier in disease (see *Tables 2.3, 2.4*).

Special points

Many of the treatments for the spondyloarthropathies were developed first for RA. They have been relatively under-researched. The development of tumour necrosis factor (TNF) inhibitors has been almost more revolutionary in the management of AS than in RA, in part because there were so few other options previously. The conventional disease modifying antirheumatic drugs (DMARDs) are not effective in spinal disease, but can be helpful in the management of the associated peripheral arthritis.

Classification criteria (Tables 2.3, 2.4)

Table 2.3 Assessment of spondyloarthritis classification criteria (ASAS) for people with back pain for 3 months or longer who were <45 years old at onset of back pain

Sacroiliitis on imaging* plus 1 or more spondyloarthritis features†

Or

HLA-B27 plus 2 or more other spondyloarthritis features†

* Sacroiliitis on imaging: active (acute) inflammation on MRI highly suggestive of sacroiliitis associated with spondyloarthritis, or definite radiographic sacroiliitis according to the modified New York criteria

† Spondyloarthritis features: inflammatory back pain; arthritis; enthesitis (heel); uveitis; dactylitis; psoriasis; Crohn's disease/ulcerative colitis; good response to NSAIDs; family history of spondyloarthritis; HLA-B27; elevated C-reactive protein

Adapted from Rudwaleit *et al*. (2009).

Table 2.4 Modified New York criteria for the diagnosis of anklylosing spondylitis

Clinical criteria:

Lower back pain; present for more than 3 months; improved by exercise but not relieved by rest

Limitation of lumbar spine motion in both the sagittal and frontal planes

Limitation of chest expansion relative to normal values for age and sex

Radiological criterion:

Sacroiliitis on x-ray*

Diagnosis:

Definite AS if the radiological criterion is present plus at least one clinical criterion

Probable AS if three clinical criteria are present alone, or if the radiological criterion is present but no clinical criteria are present

* In practice, MRI evidence of synovitis has now surpassed the use of x-ray, where available, because of its improved sensitivity.

Adapted from van der Linden *et al*. (1984).

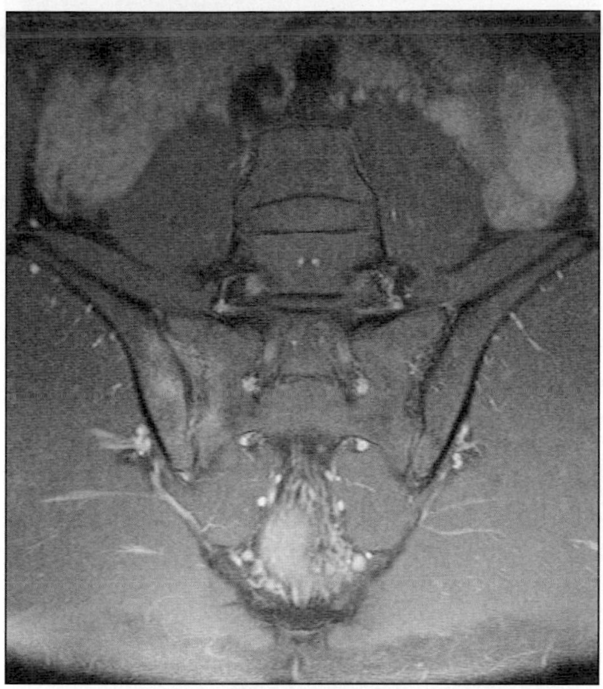

Fig. 2.9 Unilateral right sided sacroiliitis on MRI in a young man with right sided buttock pain and known ulcerative colitis.

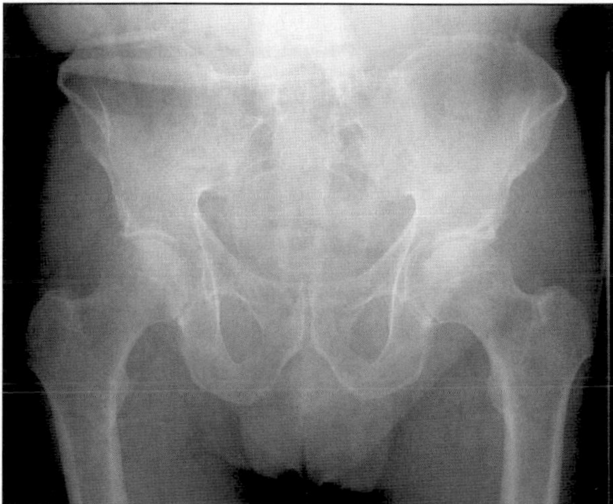

Fig. 2.10 Fused sacroiliac joints in a 40-year-old man with long-standing AS.

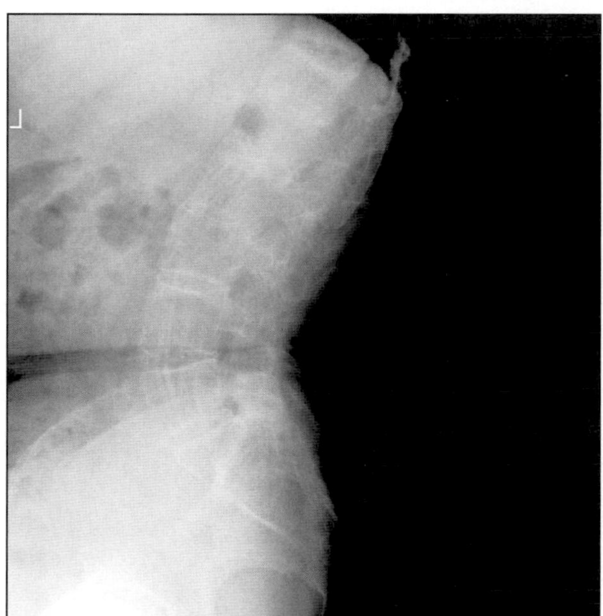

Fig. 2.11 Bamboo spine, caused by fusing syndesmophytes, seen on plain film in a man with long-standing AS. Note also the osteopenia.

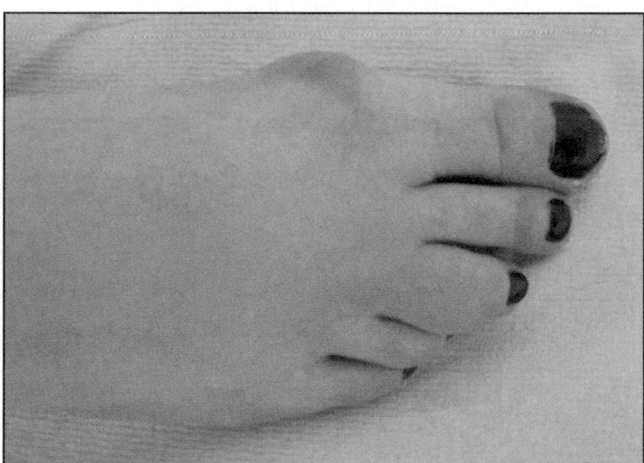

Fig. 2.12 Dactylitis of the middle toe in a young woman with psoriatic arthritis.

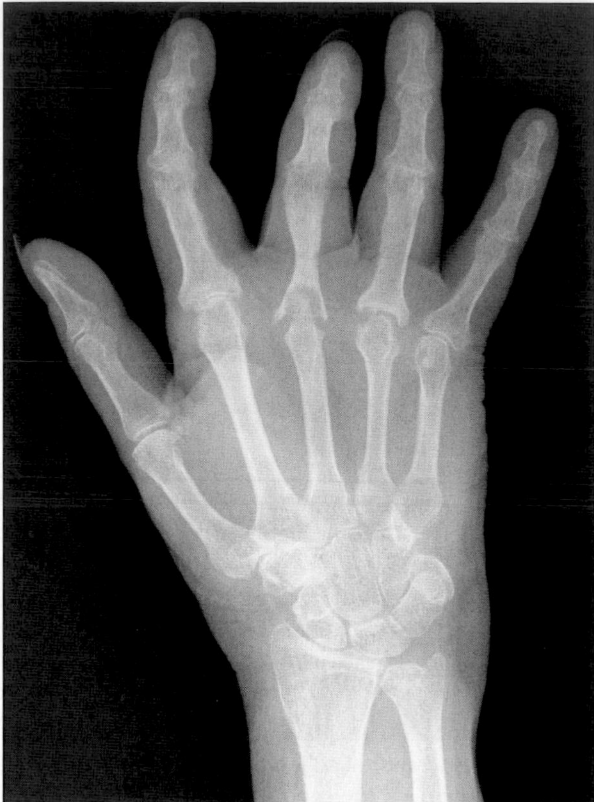

Fig. 2.13 Hand x-ray of a patient with long-standing psoriatic arthritis showing telescoping of the right middle MCP and reduction in joint space, with erosive change affecting the PIPs and DIPs.

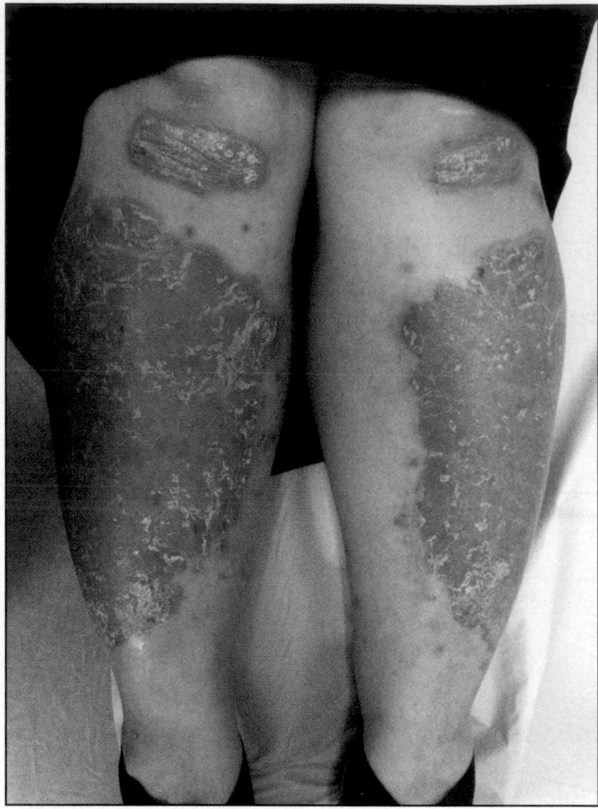

Fig. 2.14 Plaque psoriasis in a young woman.

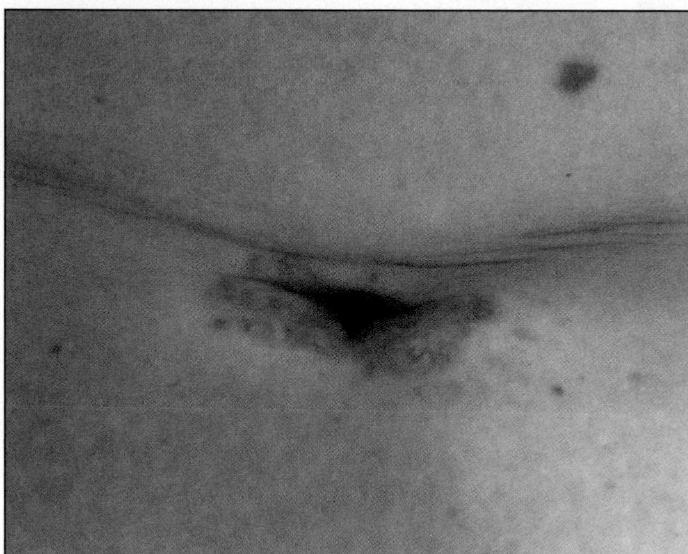

Fig. 2.15 Small patch of psoriasis around the umbilicus – a good place to look.

3 SYSTEMIC LUPUS ERYTHEMATOSUS AND THE AUTOIMMUNE RHEUMATIC DISEASES

See cases 3, 6, 13, 23, 32, 35, 37, 39, 45, 48, 51, 59, 67, 71, 76, 81, 99

Definition and clinical features

Systemic lupus erythematosus (SLE), or lupus, is a multisystem autoimmune rheumatic disease, which is associated with the presence of autoantibodies, in particular those directed against nuclear antigens. The spectrum of disease is broad, from a mild syndrome of rash, joint pain and fatigue, to a life threatening syndrome of renal failure or uncontrolled neurological disease.

Patients who meet any four of the 11 classification criteria (*Table 2.5*) are considered to have SLE; 3 criteria suggest probable SLE. New classification criteria have recently been tested by the Systemic Lupus International Collaborating Clinics, which were found to be more sensitive but less specific than the ACR criteria in identifying patients considered to have SLE by expert clinicians (Petri *et al.*, 2012).

Epidemiology

SLE affects approximately 1 in 1,000 people and is up to 10 times more common in women than men, particularly affecting those of child-bearing age. SLE is more common and severe in some ethnic groups, e.g. Black and Asian.

Table 2.5 Criteria for classification of SLE

Criterion	Definition/examples
1 Malar rash	Fixed erythema over the malar eminences, tending to spare the nasolabial folds
2 Discoid rash	Erythematous raised patches, may scar
3 Photosensitivity	Skin rash as a result of unusual reaction to sunlight
4 Oral ulcers	Usually painless
5 Arthritis	Often non-erosive (e.g. Jaccoud's arthropathy)
6 Serositis	a Pleuritis – pleuritic pain, pleural rub, pleural effusion b Pericarditis – ECG changes, rub, pericardial effusion
7 Renal disorder	a Proteinuria (>3+ or 0.5 g/day) b Cellular casts in urine
8 Neurological disorder*	a Seizures b Psychosis
9 Haematological disorder	a Haemolytic anaemia b Leucopenia c Lymphopenia d Thrombocytopenia
10 Immunological disorder	a Anti-dsDNA antibodies b Anti-Sm antibodies c Anti-phospholipid antibodies
11 Anti-nuclear antibody	Exclude drug causes

* The list of possible neurological manifestations of SLE has since been extended by the ACR (1999).

Adapted from Tan *et al.* (1982); and Hochberg (1997).

Differential diagnosis

The differential in autoimmune rheumatic disease is very broad, depending upon which disease manifestations are noted (see *Table 2.6*).

It is important to exclude infections, in particular bacterial endocarditis, human immunodeficiency virus (HIV) and tuberculosis (TB), all of which can cause multisystem disease. Some drugs can cause lupus-like syndromes, including procainamide and hydralazine, but disease is usually relatively mild, with renal involvement seen very rarely. TNF inhibitors commonly cause the development of new ANAs, but very seldom cause actual drug induced lupus.

There is also significant overlap with other autoimmune rheumatic diseases.

Investigations

SLE is almost always associated with a positive ANA, and its absence should make you suspicious about the diagnosis. Often other autoantibodies are seen, with varying specificity, sensitivity and disease associations, e.g. anti-double stranded deoxyribonucleic acid (anti-dsDNA) antibodies are highly specific and associated with renal disease.

Active disease is also associated with a high ESR, low complement and lymphopenia. Anaemia and thrombocytopenia are also commonly seen.

Urinalysis, renal function and blood pressure should be checked at each visit because of the risks associated with untreated renal involvement.

Special points

Autoimmune conditions frequently 'hunt in packs', so patients should be screened for associated conditions, such as thyroid disease, Sjögren's syndrome and anti-phospholipid syndrome. Unlike the erythrocyte sedimentatiom rate (ESR), the C-reactive protein (CRP) is often normal in patients with SLE. A high CRP should prompt investigations for a coexisting infection, but is also seen in patients with active arthritis and serositis.

Table 2.6 Differential diagnosis – features and investigations

Condition	Clinical features	Key investigations
Sjögren's syndrome	Dry eyes and mouth (sicca) Arthralgia Fatigue Increased risk of lymphoma	ANA Ro and La Lip biopsy
Anti-phospholipid syndrome	Arterial and/or venous thromboembolism Pregnancy morbidity Livedo reticularis	Positive anti-cardiolipin antibodies or lupus anticoagulant
Systemic sclerosis	Raynaud's phenomenon Scleroderma Sclerodactyly Pulmonary fibrosis Renal crisis	ANA Scl-70/anti-centromere antibodies
Polymyositis and dermatomyositis (DM)	Proximal muscle weakness Characteristic rash in DM – Gottron's papules on knuckles, heliotrope rash on face, erythroderma	CK levels ANA and anti-synthetase antibodies EMG MRI muscles Muscle and skin biopsy Investigation for underlying malignancy, particularly in DM

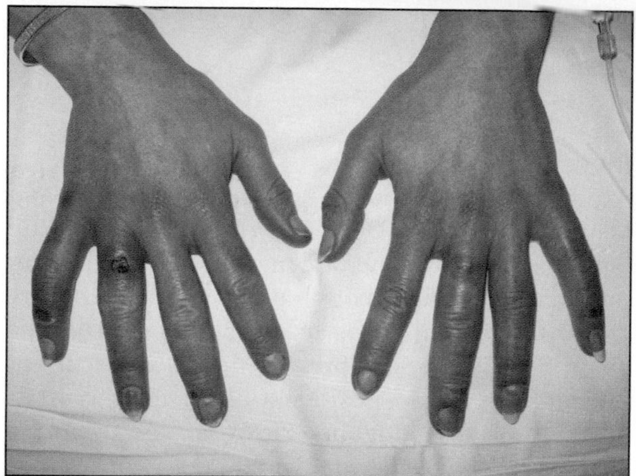

Fig. 2.16 Raynaud's phenomenon with ulceration in a young woman with primary Raynaud's disease. She was receiving IV prostacyclin (iloprost) because of severity of symptoms and ulceration, which is rare in primary disease.

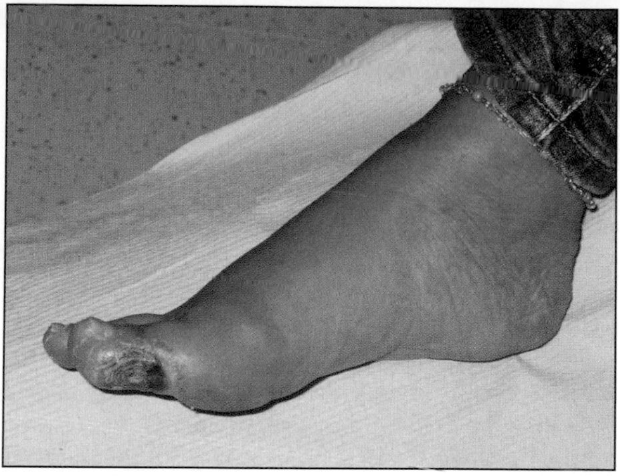

Fig. 2.17 A vasculitic ulcer on the toe of a 40-year-old woman with SLE.

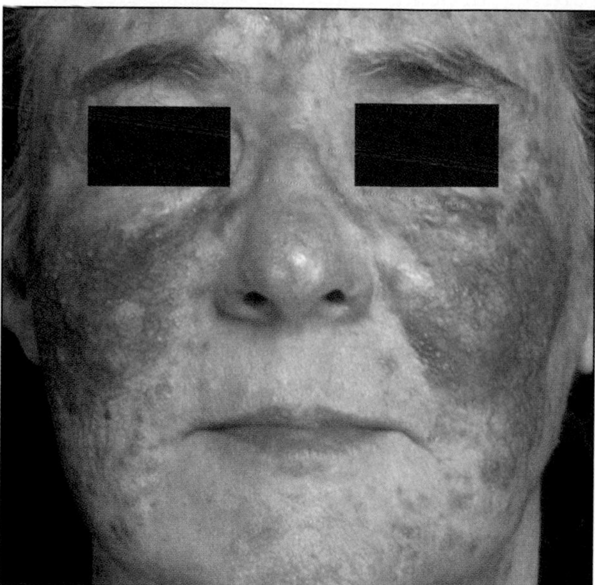

Fig. 2.18 The typical butterfly facial rash of SLE; note the relative sparing of the nasolabial folds. (Courtesy of St John's Institute of Dermatology [King's College], Guy's Hospital, London; from: Rycroft *et al.* [2010] *Dermatology, a Colour Handbook*, CRC Press.)

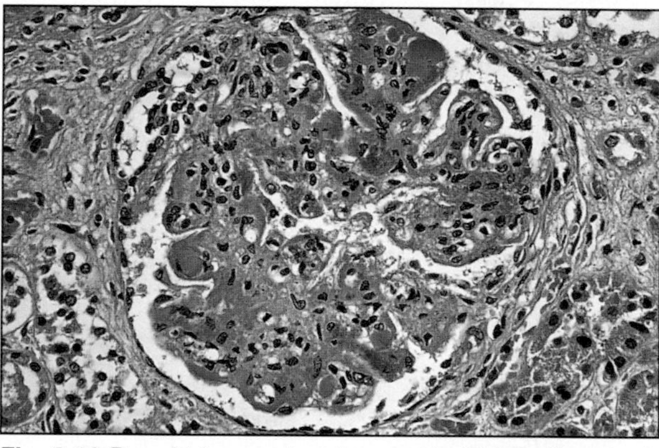

Fig. 2.19 Renal biopsy showing grade IV (proliferative) lupus nephritis. (Courtesy of Pattison *et al.* [2004] *Renal Medicine, a Colour Handbook*, CRC Press.)

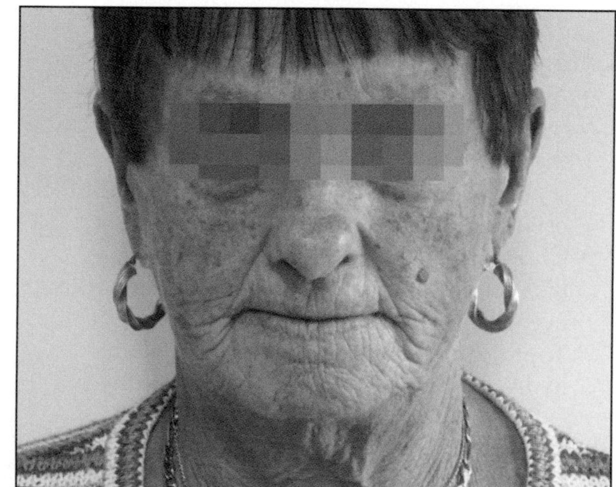

Fig. 2.20 A 74-year-old woman with limited cutaneous systemic sclerosis; note telangiectasia, tightening of skin around the nose, and beaking of the mouth.

4 CRYSTAL ARTHROPATHIES

See cases 7, 40, 43, 74

Definition and clinical features

There are two main types of crystal arthropathy, gout and pseudogout. Gout describes the clinical syndromes associated with the inflammatory response to the deposition of monosodium urate (MSU) crystals. Acute gout refers to episodes of inflammatory mono- or oligoarticular arthritis, which typically involve the first metatarsophalangeal (MTP) joint of the great toe (podagra), and/or the ankle or knee. Onset is abrupt and the pain is very severe. The joint is hot and swollen and the overlying skin may peel. Even without treatment, at least in early disease, attacks are usually self-limiting, and resolve within about 7 days.

Chronic tophaceous gout refers to the deposition of solid MSU crystals within the joints, causing a chronic, destructive inflammatory arthritis, and tophi in the subcutaneous tissues – classically the pinnae of the ear, but also around the elbows, and within the Achilles tendon and finger tip pulp.

Pseudogout resembles acute gout in clinical presentation, but occurs more commonly in women, affects joints in a different order of frequency (knee, shoulder and wrist), and is caused by calcium pyrophosphate crystals.

Epidemiology

Overall prevalence of gout was approximately 1% in the UK and USA, but is now increasing dramatically. It is about five times more common in men than women, and the primary condition is essentially not seen in premenopausal women. By contrast, pseudogout is more common in women than men.

Differential diagnosis

- Acute gout: recurrent podagra has no true mimics, but in all other situations, the important differential diagnosis is a septic arthritis. Other differentials include pseudogout and a reactive arthritis.
- Chronic tophaceous gout: RA is the main differential, though there is actually a striking negative association between RA and gout. Tophi can be confused with the calcium hydroxyapatite deposits seen in scleroderma.

Investigations

Aspiration of a joint, bursa or tophus and identification of MSU crystals (which are visible on light microscopy, and are negatively birefringent on polarizing microscopy) allow for the definitive diagnosis of gout to be made, and is appropriate apart from when the presentation is of recurrent podagra. Similarly, positively birefringent crystals are seen in pseudogout. However, the reported absence of crystals in an aspirate does not exclude the diagnosis, as they can be missed.

Typically during an acute attack, crystals can be seen within phagocytosing macrophages and neutrophils. The identification of high uric acid levels in blood, although commonly found, can be misleading, and is only relevant if it fits the clinical pattern. An acute attack can be associated with a fall in uric acid levels. Acute gout is accompanied by an often dramatic rise in inflammatory markers, and sometimes a modest neutrophilia.

Deposition of tophi within a joint causes an erosive arthropathy. On x-ray, erosions have well demarcated, sclerotic edges, and appear 'punched out'.

Special points

Serum uric acid levels increase with age, male sex, obesity, high alcohol intake, hypertension and a purine rich diet. In addition hyperuricaemia is seen with some drug treatment, particularly diuretics, and during the treatment of cancer, particularly the haematological malignancies. In most situations however, asymptomatic hyperuricaemia does not need to be treated. Similarly, asymptomatic chondrocalcinosis is often seen on plain films but in itself doesn't require particular treatment.

Importantly, the joint aspirate in an acute crystal arthropathy can look just like frank pus, as is expected in a septic arthritis. Aspiration and microscopy/culture of synovial fluid is therefore crucial for diagnosis. If in doubt, treat for sepsis first until the cultures become available.

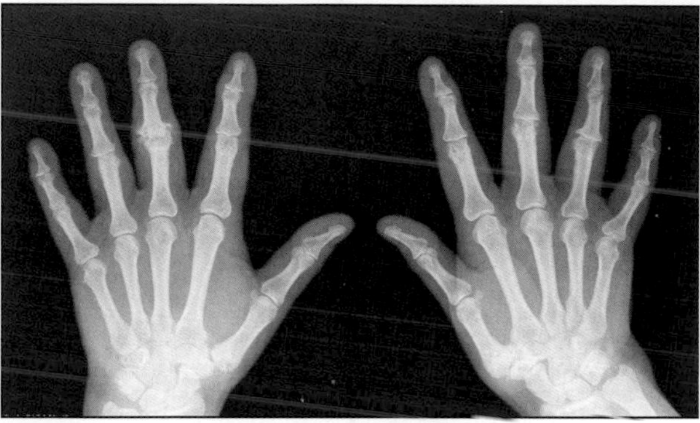

Fig. 2.21 Coexisting OA and chronic gout in a 74-year-old man. Note the destruction of the left middle finger PIP with small punched out erosions. There is also an erosion affecting the PIP of the right finger. Other joints demonstrate predominant OA change, e.g. sclerosis, joint space narrowing and osteophyte narrowing in the right ring finger PIP.

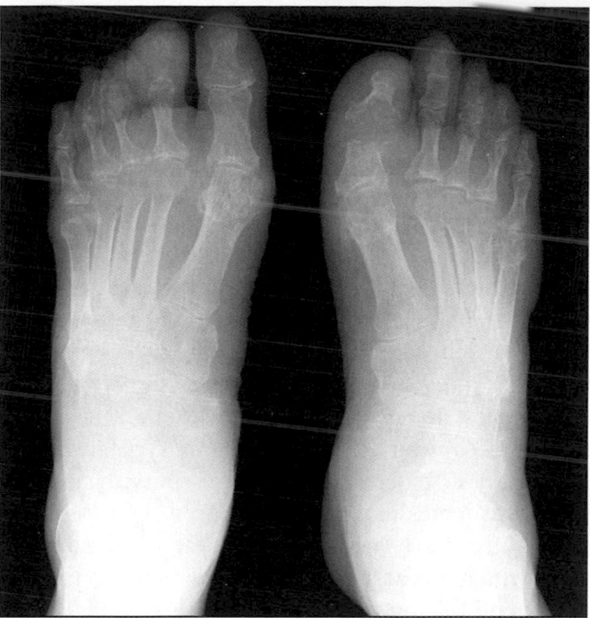

Fig. 2.22 X-ray of feet of a patient with chronic tophaceous gout. Note the complete destruction of the interphalangeal joint of the right great toe, with the joint being replaced by gouty tophus.

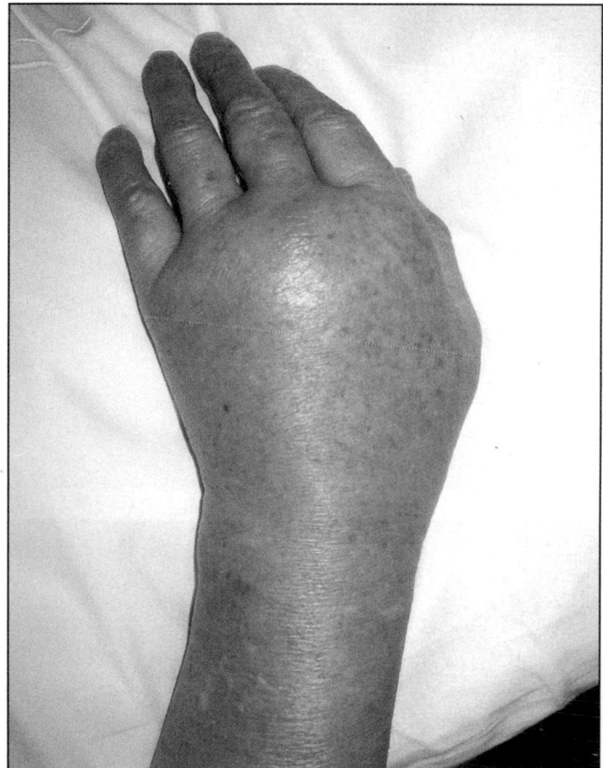

Fig. 2.23 A 68-year-old woman with acute onset pain and swelling of the left wrist. Aspirate confirmed the presence of calcium pyrophosphate crystals.

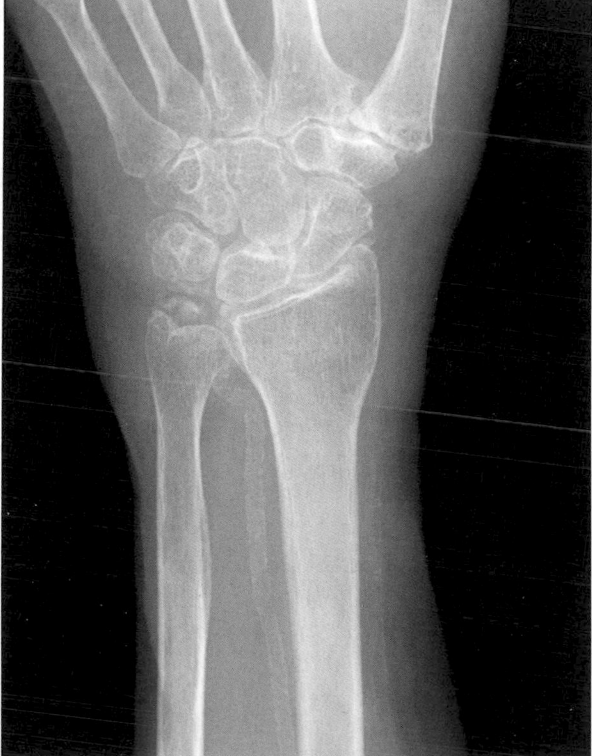

Fig. 2.24 Calcification of the triangular cartilage shown on x-ray of an elderly woman presenting with an acutely swollen wrist with aspirate proven pseudogout. Also note the changes of first CMC OA.

5 VASCULITIDES, INCLUDING GIANT CELL ARTERITIS AND POLYMYALGIA RHEUMATICA

See cases 8, 22, 34, 56

Definition and clinical features

This group of conditions encompasses a variety of disorders clustered together because of their underlying pathology – inflammation in the wall of blood vessels, predominantly arteries. They can be further subdivided on the basis of the size of the artery they affect (*Table 2.7*). Although, as listed, there are clinical features which are typical of each condition, in general they also present with systemic features such as malaise, fever and weight loss.

Giant cell arteritis and polymyalgia rheumatica, with which it is associated, are dealt with separately at the end of this section.

Epidemiology

The most common condition is giant cell arteritis, affecting 1 in 500 adults over age 50 years. The anti-neutrophil cytoplasmic antibody (ANCA) associated vasculitides have an annual incidence of about 10 per million in the UK.

Differential diagnosis

- Small vessel vasculitis associated with infections, particularly viruses
- Small vessel vasculitis associated with other autoimmune rheumatic diseases, particularly SLE
- Paraneoplastic phenomena.

Investigations

- Biopsy
- ANCA.

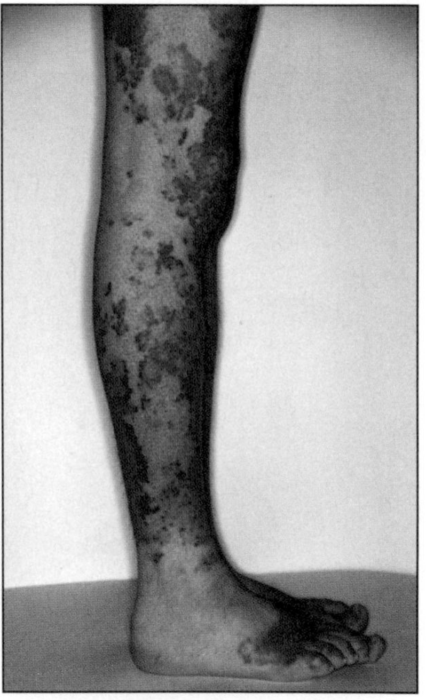

Fig. 2.25 Palpable purpura on the legs of a 50-year-old woman.

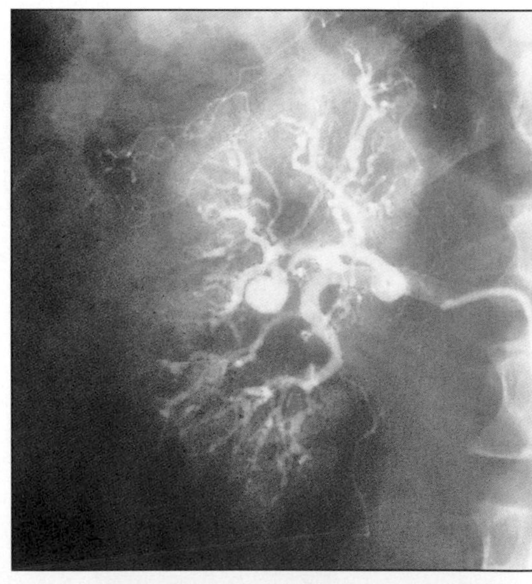

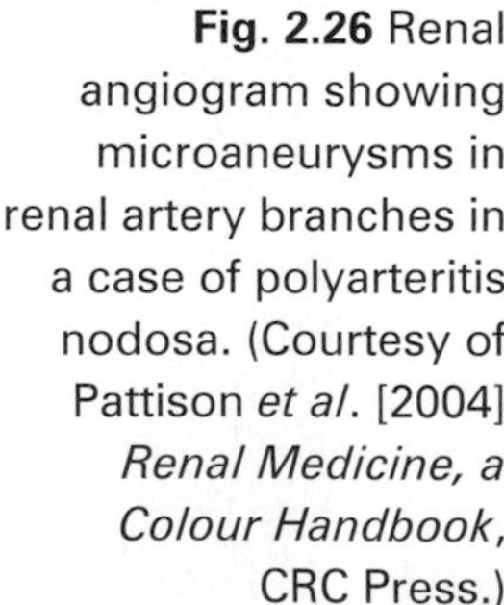

Fig. 2.26 Renal angiogram showing microaneurysms in renal artery branches in a case of polyarteritis nodosa. (Courtesy of Pattison *et al.* [2004] *Renal Medicine, a Colour Handbook*, CRC Press.)

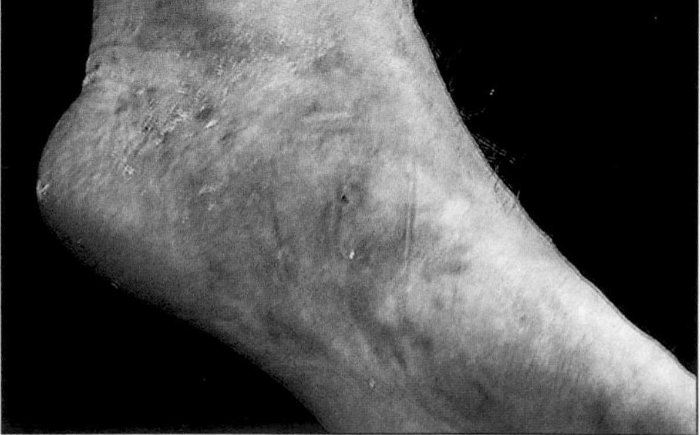

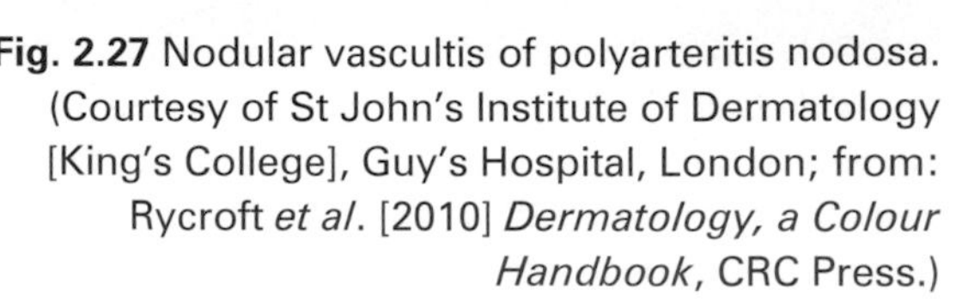

Fig. 2.27 Nodular vascultis of polyarteritis nodosa. (Courtesy of St John's Institute of Dermatology [King's College], Guy's Hospital, London; from: Rycroft *et al.* [2010] *Dermatology, a Colour Handbook*, CRC Press.)

Table 2.7 Classification of vasculitides according to size of artery affected

Artery size	Condition	Peak age	Clinical presentation	Diagnosis
Large	Giant cell arteritis/ polymyalgia rheumatica (see later section)	Over 50 years	Temporal headache Jaw claudication Shoulder and hip girdle stiffness	Temporal artery biopsy Clinical picture and response to steroids
	Takayasu's arteritis	10–40 years	Systemic features Asymmetric pulses Claudication	Angiographic evidence of stenosis
Medium	Polyarteritis nodosa	Increases with age	Systemic upset Renal failure Neurological manifestations Abdominal pain	Angiography showing aneurysms
Small including arterioles	Granulomatosis with polyangiitis (GPA, Wegener's granulomatosis)	Older adults	Nasal, lung and renal disease	ANCA associated Typically c-ANCA, anti-PR3 antibodies
	Microscopic polyangiitis	Older adults	Overlap with GPA, but absence of granuloma on biopsy	ANCA associated Typically p-ANCA, anti-MPO antibodies
	Eosinophilic granulomatosis with polyangiitis (EGPA, Churg–Strauss syndrome)	Middle age	Rhinitis Late onset asthma Neuropathy Eosinophilia	ANCA associated Typically p-ANCA, anti-MPO antibodies
	Henloch–Schönlein purpura	Childhood	Petechial rash Abdominal pain IgA-mediated renal disease	Clinical picture
Other	Behçet's disease Affects multiple sizes of vessel including veins	30–40 years	Oral and genital ulcers Rash Uveitis Arthritis	Clinical picture

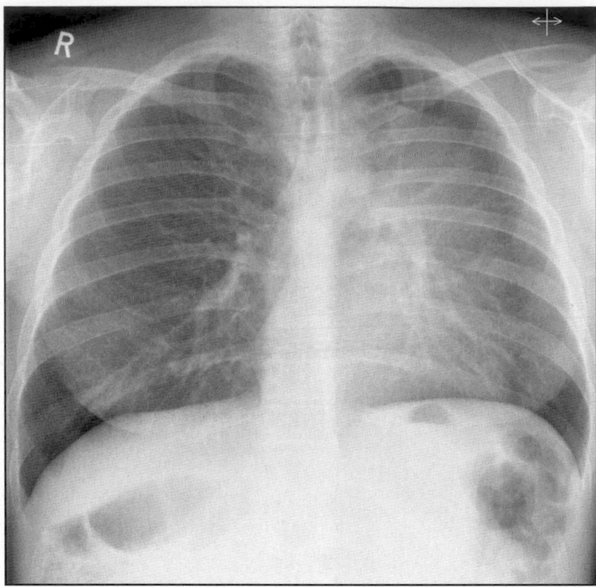

Fig. 2.28a, 2.28b Chest x-rays from a 34-year-old man presenting with fever, weight loss and deafness. Diagnosis was later confirmed as GPA (previously Wegener's granulomatosis). **2.28a** Pretreatment with cyclophosphamide; **2.28b** post-treatment. Note resolution of ring lesions, but persistence of mediastinal mass.

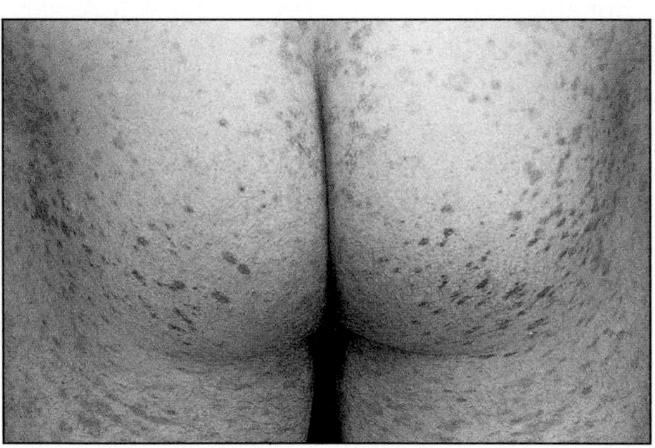

Fig. 2.29 Small vessel vasculitis due to Henoch-–Schönlein purpura showing the classical involvement of the buttocks. (Courtesy of St John's Institute of Dermatology [King's College], Guy's Hospital, London; from: Rycroft *et al*. [2010] *Dermatology, a Colour Handbook*, CRC Press.)

GIANT CELL ARTERITIS AND POLYMYALGIA RHEUMATICA

Definition and clinical features

These two conditions are closely linked, and polymyalgia rheumatica (PMR) is the more common and generally less severe of the two. In patients with a clinical syndrome suggestive of PMR, up to 20% will have coexistent giant cell arteritis (GCA), and in patients with GCA, up to 50% will report symptoms of PMR.

PMR causes muscle stiffness and pain around the hip and shoulder girdles, associated with fatigue and malaise, and raised inflammatory markers. Muscle strength is preserved. When severe, stiffness, particularly in the morning, can be incapacitating, and systemic features such as weight loss and fever can be seen. GCA, or temporal arteritis, is a large vessel vasculitis which causes temporal headache, jaw claudication, visual disturbance and the risk of blindness or stroke. Again, systemic features can be dominant, with some patients presenting as though they had a malignancy.

Rapid response to steroids is the key to both diagnoses, and the absence of this response should lead you to question the diagnosis.

Epidemiology

Both conditions are rare in non-White populations and are approximately twice as common in women as men. The disease frequency increases with age, and both are very rare under the age of 50 years.

Differential diagnosis

- Malignancy
- Subacute infection such as TB, bacterial endocarditis
- The myalgic presentation of RA – not uncommon in an older population.

Investigations

Raised inflammatory markers are key to the diagnosis. Although cases with normal ESR/CRP are described, these are rare. Anaemia is also seen.

Temporal artery biopsy remains the gold standard for diagnosis of GCA. A normal biopsy does not exclude GCA however, as the inflammatory changes are known to exist as skip lesions, i.e. patches of vasculitic change interspersed with patches of normal artery. Increasingly, non-invasive tests such as ultrasound and positron emission tomography (PET) are being used.

Special points

Investigations should not delay treatment in GCA because of the risk of blindness. High doses of steroids should be prescribed immediately for those considered at risk.

Remember the population you are treating – long-term steroids in the elderly carry a significant risk and bone and gastroprotection should be considered.

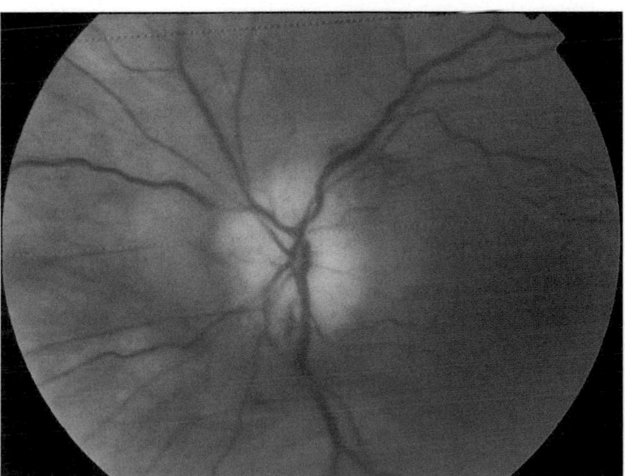

Fig. 2.30 Ischaemic optic neuritis in a patient with giant cell arteritis. (Courtesy of Mr Fion Bremnar, Consulant Ophthalmologist, University College Hospital.)

6 OSTEOARTHRITIS

See cases 47, 54, 58

Definition and clinical features

The most common symptom in osteoarthritis (OA) is pain, which is insidious in onset. Unlike the inflammatory arthritides, pain tends to be worse after use, and although patients may complain of early morning stiffness, this usually lasts less than 30 minutes. OA can affect virtually every joint in the body, but it most commonly involves the hands, feet, hips and knees. Typically the symptoms, if not the signs, are asymmetric.

On examination, joints may be swollen due to bony enlargement, synovitis or an effusion. The joints are usually cool (even in the presence of an effusion) and the overlying skin not erythematous. Range of movement may be limited, and movement may be associated with crepitus.

Different patterns of joint disease have been recognized. Nodal disease involving the distal (Heberden's nodes) and/or proximal (Bouchard's nodes) interphalangeal (IP) joints is more common in women, and tends to run in families. Patients often complain that the joints are unsightly and tender, rather than severely painful. First carpometacarpal (CMC) pain is also common and can cause quite disabling pain, but this usually settles over a few years. Hip and knee OA tend to affect different people, and can significantly impact mobility, requiring joint replacement surgery. Knee OA is associated with valgus or varus deformity.

Epidemiology

OA is extremely common, though there is a discrepancy between the radiological and the clinical diagnosis. There are known genetic associations, and the incidence of OA is increased by some systemic factors such as obesity but also due to local factors such as trauma or overuse.

Differential diagnosis

Some patients go through an inflammatory phase, where the symptoms can be confused for an inflammatory arthritis. On the whole, however, the pattern of disease and the symptoms make the diagnosis quite clear.

Investigations

All blood tests including inflammatory markers should be normal, though there is an association with other conditions such as diabetes and haemochromatosis. In addition, in the older age group with possible multiple pathologies, blood tests may be abnormal for unrelated reasons.

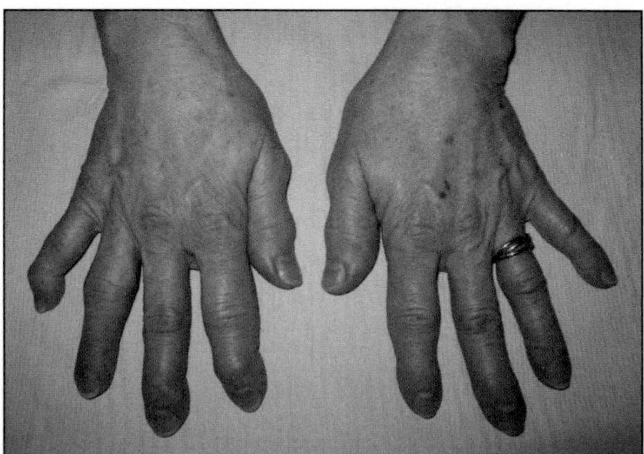

Fig. 2.31 Nodal OA hands, showing Heberden's nodes, especially affecting the right hand, and Bouchard's nodes affecting both index fingers, and the right ring finger.

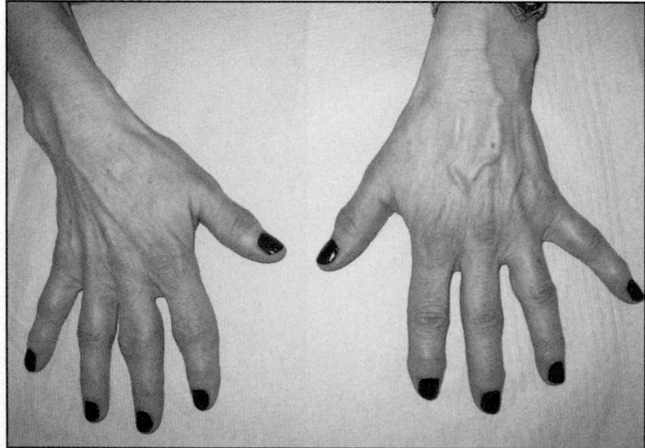

Fig. 2.32 Bouchard's nodes affecting middle and index finger of the right hand.

Features of OA visible on plain radiographs include loss of joint space, which is typically asymmetrical, subchondral sclerosis and bone cysts and osteophytosis.

Special points

Currently, the management of OA is based on symptom control, with analgesia and physiotherapy used in the early stages, and surgical intervention considered when symptoms become too severe. Research in OA is now blossoming, with a hope that disease modifying drugs will be developed in due course.

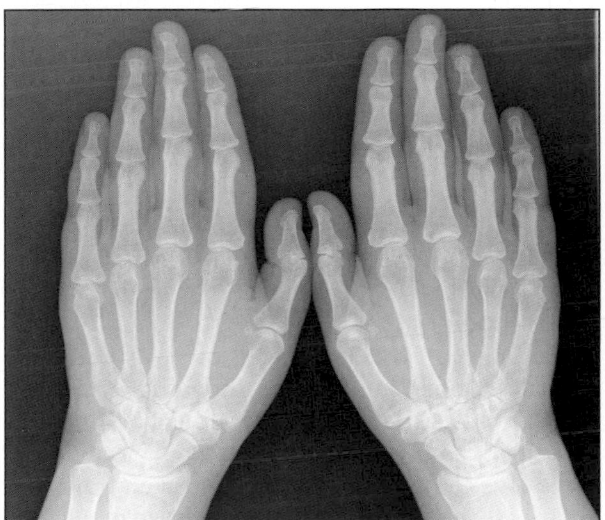

Fig. 2.33 Plain x-ray showing erosive OA of the left first CMC joint. The first CMCs are almost exclusively affected by OA.

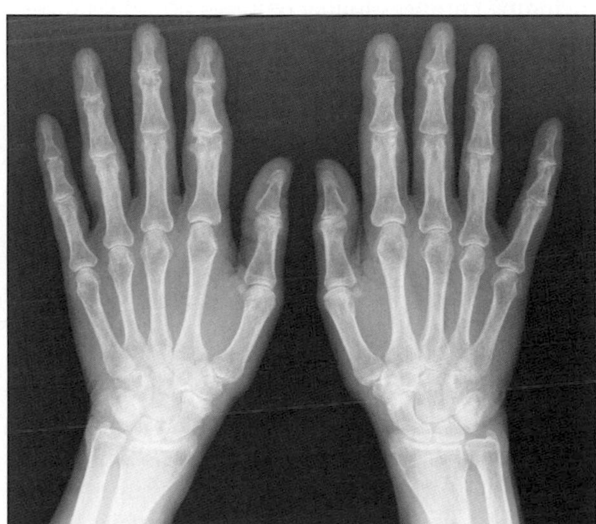

Fig. 2.34 Plain x-ray of the patient in **2.31** showing nodal osteoarthritis – reduced joint space, cyst formation and osteophytes affecting the DIP and the PIP joints, particularly in both index fingers. Note also surrounding soft tissue swelling.

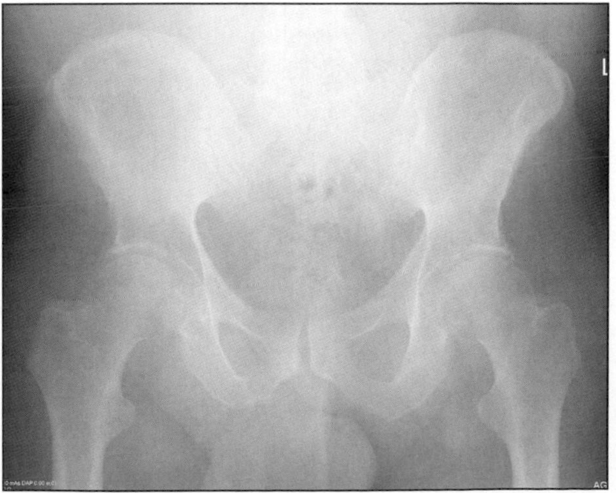

Fig. 2.35 Plain x-ray showing OA of the hips – loss of joint space and osteophyte formation on the left.

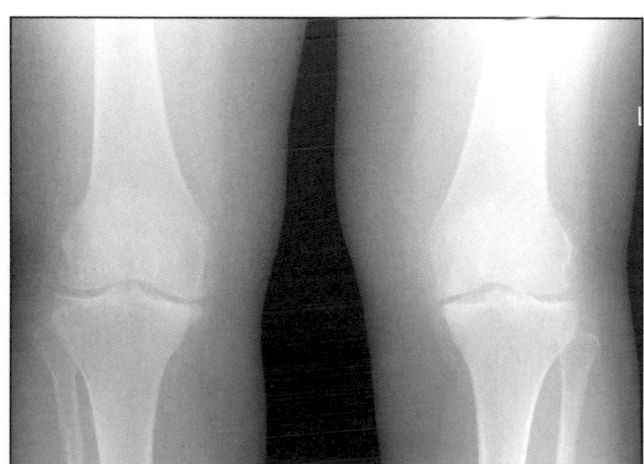

Fig. 2.36 Plain x-ray showing OA of the knees – loss of joint space especially medially, with osteophyte formation.

7 CHRONIC WIDESPREAD PAIN/ FIBROMYALGIA

See case 27

Definition and clinical features

The terminology here is difficult because it is inconsistent and sometimes controversial. Most of the controversy surrounds whether fibromyalgia exists as a discrete condition, or as part of a more general group of medically unexplained syndromes including chronic fatigue, irritable bowel syndrome and non-cardiac chest pain. Chronic widespread pain is generally defined as pain for greater than 3 months involving the left and right side of the body, and both above and below the waist. Fibromyalgia combines this clinical presentation with at least 11 out of 18 tender trigger points (**Figure 2.37**). In almost all patients there are other associated features, often the most important of which are poor sleep and mood disturbance, and also include numbness, paraesthesia and morning stiffness.

Epidemiology

Prevalence of chronic widespread pain is thought to be up to 10% in Western populations with about 5% fulfilling the criteria for fibromyalgia. These conditions are more common in women, with a peak in those aged 50–75 years. Fibromyalgia in particular has been shown to be common in patients with other rheumatological conditions, in particular SLE and Sjögren's syndrome.

Differential diagnosis

This is really about exclusion. Before making the diagnosis, you have to be confident that the patient doesn't have another cause of musculoskeletal pain including:

- Inflammatory arthritis
- Autoimmune rheumatic diseases
- PMR
- Hypo/hypercalcaemia
- Malignancy.

Investigations

This is a clinical diagnosis. There are no investigations which support the diagnosis, but it may be appropriate to screen inflammatory markers, calcium and vitamin D and autoantibodies.

Special points

Management of these patients is complex and often difficult. People can become very disaffected and socially isolated. The doctor–patient rapport is particularly important and many people feel judged. Some drugs have been shown to be useful (tramadol, amitriptyline, gabapentin), but the roles of exercise and cognitive behavioural therapy are key.

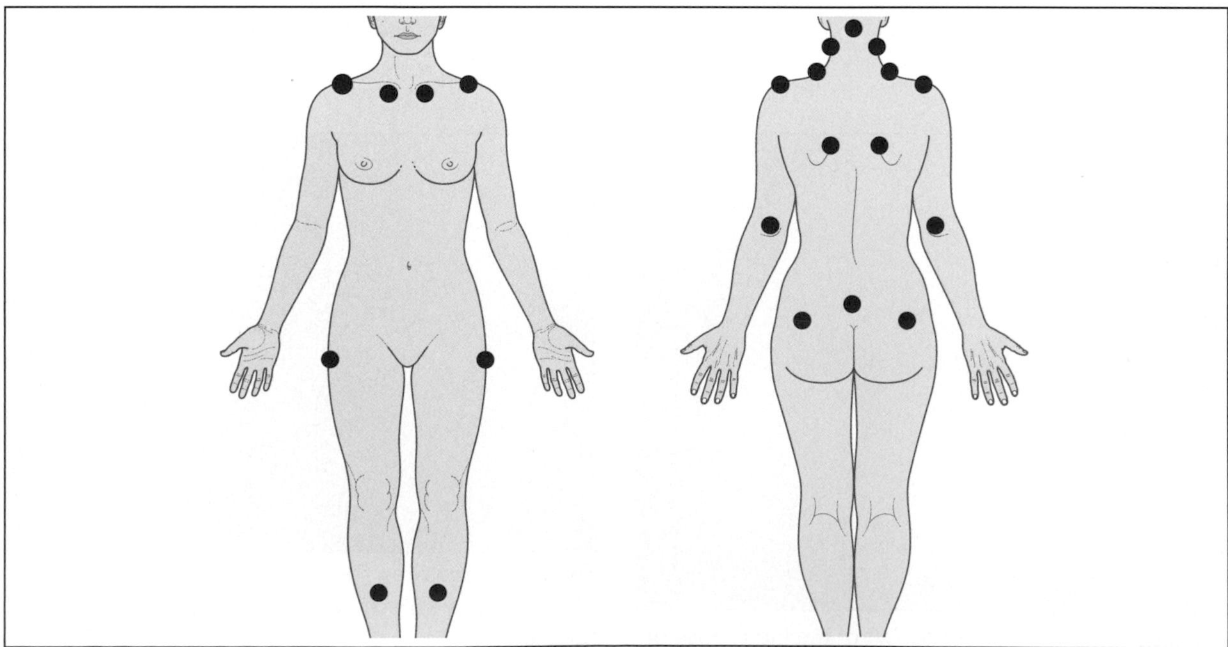

Fig. 2.37 Fibromyalgia trigger points.

8 BACK PAIN AND OTHER REGIONAL SOFT TISSUE DISORDERS

BACK PAIN

See cases 2, 17, 19, 24, 50, 65, 90, 94, 98, 100

Definition and clinical features

Clearly, back pain is not a diagnosis, it is a symptom. The vast majority of patients with back pain will have a mechanical, often muscular, cause of their symptoms (see *Table 2.8*). The first job of the assessing doctor/physiotherapist is to spot the more serious pathology, often easier said than done. Lists of so-called red and yellow flags have been created in order to try and aid that process (see *Tables 2.9* and *2.10*). Red flags suggest a more sinister pathology, and yellow flags suggest a significant psychological impact, both of which need to be pursued. On the whole, severity of pain is not helpful because of its subjectivity.

Examination is often normal, even in the presence of significant pathology. Any neurological symptoms should prompt a neurological examination. Compression of the spinal cord or cauda equina, from any cause, are neurosurgical emergencies and clinical suspicion should prompt urgent MRI and referral.

Table 2.8 Causes of back pain

Underlying pathology	Distinguishing clinical features	Key investigations
Muscular/ soft tissue	Worse when standing, walking Muscular tenderness	None
Disc prolapse and degeneration	Prolapse can cause sudden onset pain with sciatica Worse with standing, bending	Plain film can show reduced disc height MRI required to visualize discs/ nerve roots/cord
Facet joint degeneration	Gradual onset Worse with standing, walking, straightening from bending Rotation painful Radiation into buttocks	Sclerosis can be seen on plain film MRI required to visualize relationship to discs/cord/nerve roots
Osteoporotic insufficiency fracture	Can be sudden onset Loss of height Known osteoporosis	Wedge fractures visible on plain films
Spondyloarthropathy	Night pain and morning stiffness Buttock pain Other associated features, e.g. psoriasis, uveitis	Evidence of sacroiliitis on imaging Not excluded by normal inflammatory markers
Malignancy (Myeloma, secondaries)	Night pain Weight loss Systemic features Past history of malignancy	Vertebral fracture on imaging Myeloma screen Isotope bone scan in metastatic disease
Infection (Disc, bone)	Night pain Weight loss Fever Risk factors, e.g. TB, IV drug use	Plain film can be normal in discitis, MRI required Blood tests including inflammatory markers, cultures Sites of infection elsewhere

Epidemiology

Mechanical lower back pain affects over 50% of people in the UK at one time or another, the skill therefore is to know which patients require more specialist input.

Special points

In the acute setting don't forget non-spinal causes of pain such as an abdominal aortic aneurysm or pancreatitis.

Red flags should raise suspicion about a serious underlying pathology (see *Table 2.9*).

Yellow flags are psychological factors that suggest increased risk of chronicity and disability (see *Table 2.10*)

Dermatomes

Full neurological examination including dermatomes will help you to establish the level of a disc prolapse with secondary nerve impingement.

Table 2.9 Red flags indicating underlying pathology of back pain

Age under 20 or over 55 years
Systemic features, e.g. weight loss, fever
Persistent night pain
Saddle anaesthesia/sphincter disturbance
Relevant medical history – malignancy, HIV, TB, steroid use
Abnormal neurology
Thoracic pain

Table 2.10 Yellow flags indicating psychological impact of back pain

Anxiety about disabling effect of back pain
Avoidance behaviour and reduced activity
Depression, social isolation
Desire for passive rather than active treatment
Social or financial problems

EXAMPLES OF OTHER COMMON REGIONAL SOFT TISSUE DISORDERS

See cases 4, 14, 21, 29, 53, 63, 70, 72, 77, 79, 95, Table 2.11

The mainstay of treatment here is physiotherapy. There is also a role for the use of NSAIDs and in some cases, local corticosteroid injection. Occasionally, surgery is indicated.

Remember: Many of these disorders are seen more commonly in people with inflammatory rheumatological diseases.

Table 2.11 Regional soft tissue disorders

Region	Condition (description where appropriate)	Clinical features
Hand/wrist	Trigger finger (stenosing tenosynovitis of finger flexor tendons)	Finger locked in flexion with sudden release (triggering), often worse in morning Tender nodule often palpable in tendon sheath
	De Quervain's tenosynovitis (tenosynovitis of abductor pollicus longus and extensor pollicus brevis)	Pain radial aspect of wrist and base of thumb, worse on lifting with thumb abducted Made worse by making a fist, with thumb inside and passively adducting to put pressure on tendons
	Carpal tunnel syndrome (compression of median nerve at the wrist)	Pain, paraesthesia and numbness in distribution of median nerve, often worse at night; muscle wasting with loss of thenar eminence noted in severe, long-standing disease
Elbow	Olecranon bursitis	Painful, fluctuant, swelling of olecranon bursa
	Medial and lateral epicondylitis	Pain on use of elbow, especially when gripping or carrying with arm outstretched Tender at insertion point
	Rotator cuff tendonosis +/– subacromial bursitis	Pain and reduced range of movement in shoulder, pain often extends into upper arm, discomfort when lying on the shoulder at night; positive impingement tests
	Biceps tendonosis	Often accompanies rotator cuff tendonosis, causing anterior shoulder pain particularly when elbow is flexed
Hip	Trochanteric bursitis	Pain lateral aspect of thigh, with tenderness on palpation of trochanteric bursa
	Adductor tendonosis	Pain in groin with tenderness on palpation of adductor tendons
Knee	Prepatellar bursitis	Swelling over patella, usually but not always tender
	Baker's cyst (inflammation of popliteal cyst)	Swelling behind knee
Foot/ankle	Achilles tendonosis	Pain +/– swelling of the tendon, with discomfort on walking Usually mid body of tendon if non-inflammatory cause
	Tibialis posterior tendonosis	Medial ankle/foot pain, associated with loss of medial longitudinal arch
	Plantar arch collapse	Collapse of longitudinal arch causing flat foot, and secondary biomechanical foot pain
	Plantar fasciitis	Pain putting foot to the floor, especially first thing in the morning Tender over medial insertion of plantar fascia
	Morton's neuroma (entrapment of interdigital nerves between metatarsal heads)	Pain and paraesthesia in toes and tenderness in interdigital spaces

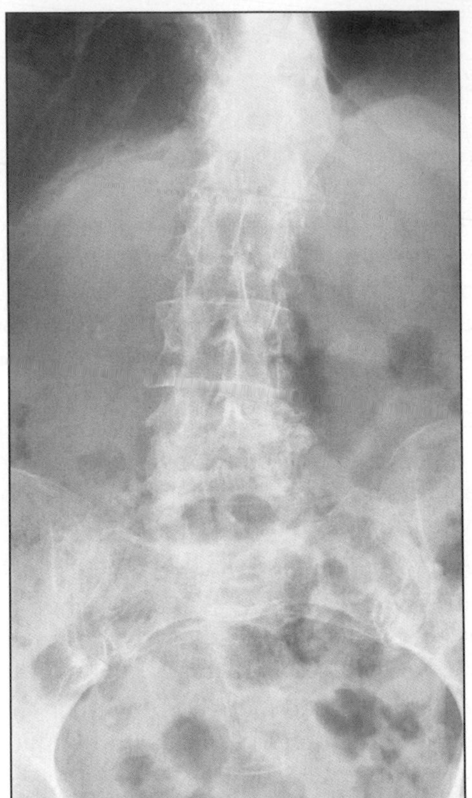

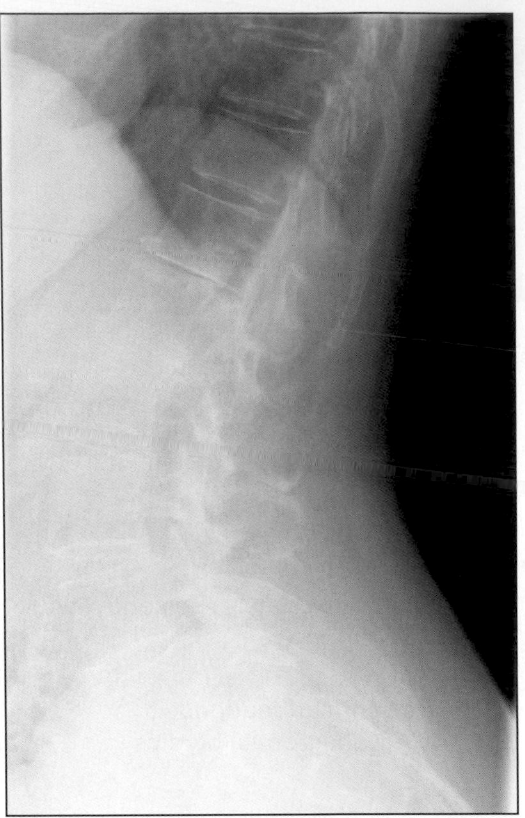

Fig. 2.38 AP (**2.38a**) and lateral (**2.38b**) plain x-rays of the lumbar spine in a middle aged lady with mechanical back pain. Advanced degenerative changes are seen, with facet joint sclerosis, reduced disc space and osteophyte formation. There is also a scoliosis.

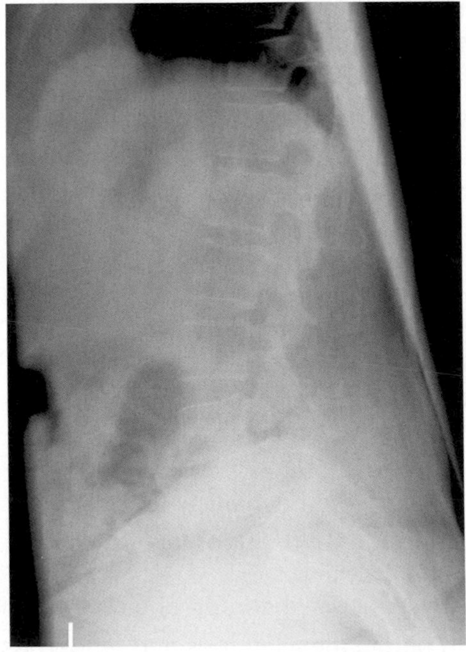

Fig. 2.39 L3/4 spondylolisthesis with pars defect – note anterior slip of the fourth on the fifth lumbar vertebra.

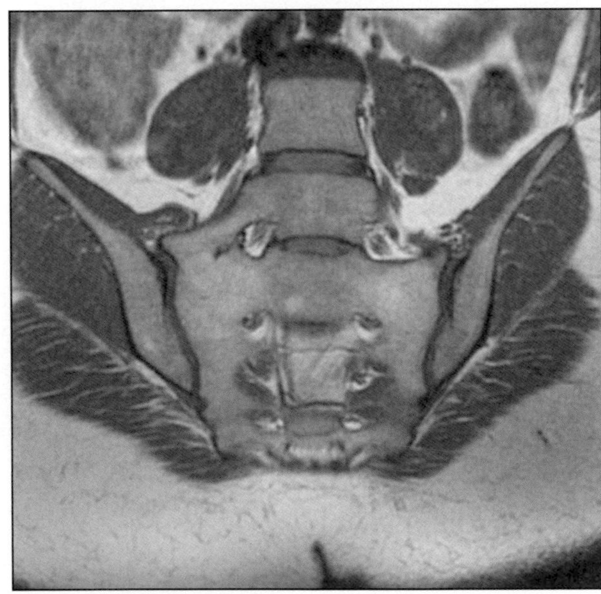

Fig. 2.40 Transitional spine on MRI – note sacralization of L5 vertebra on the right. This is thought to cause mechanical lower back pain, and an increased risk of herniation of the disc at the level above.

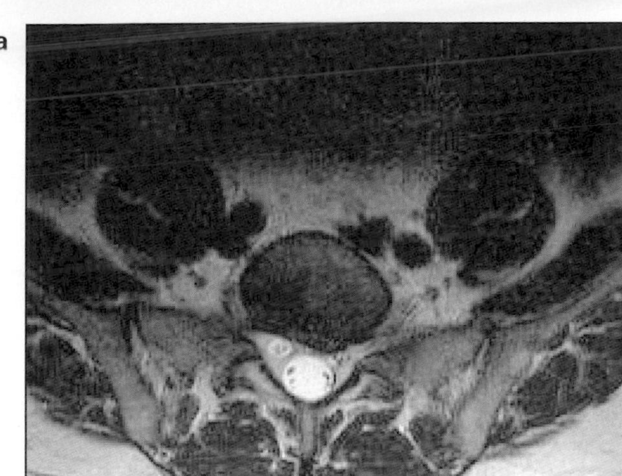

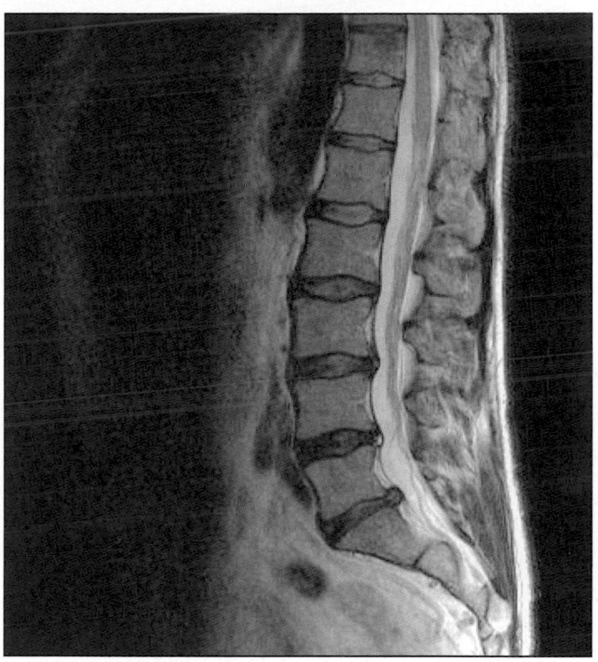

Fig. 2.41 Transverse (**2.41a**) and sagittal (**2.41b**) T2-weighted MRI image of herniated lumbosacral disc, with compression of the exiting nerve root.

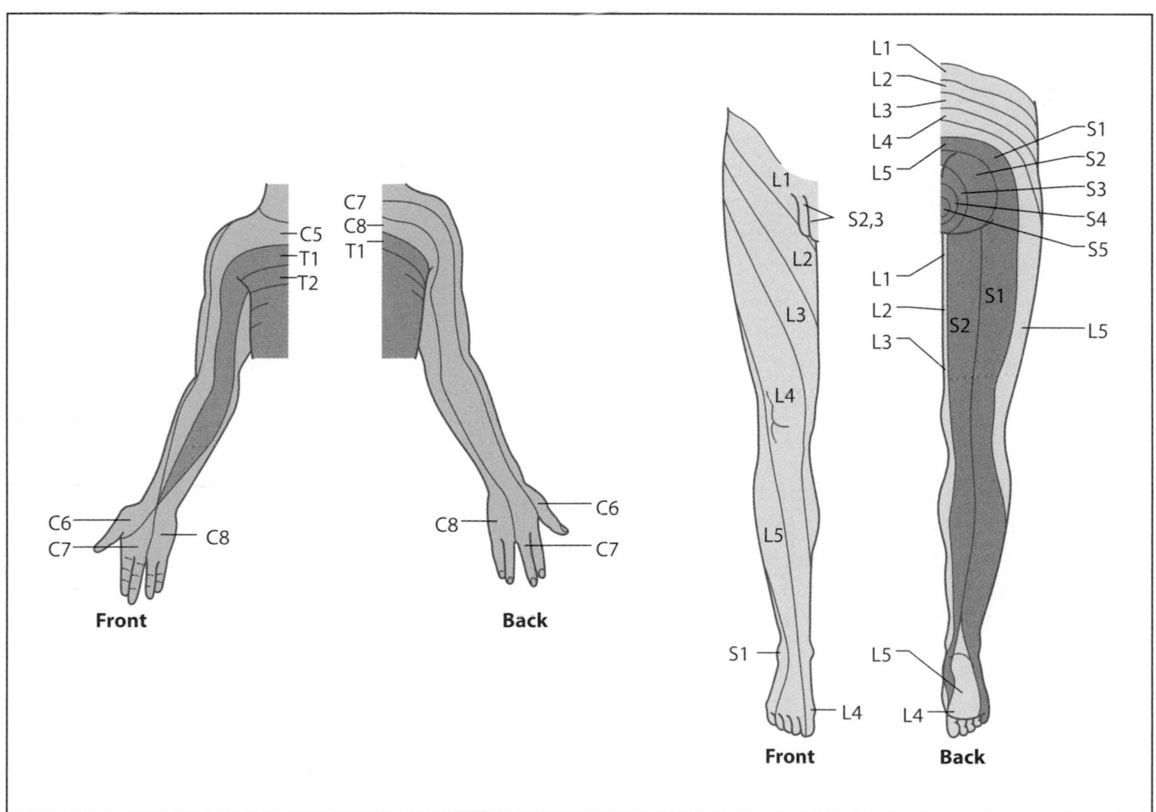

Fig. 2.42 Distribution of the cervical and thoracic dermatomes.

9 OSTEOPOROSIS AND METABOLIC BONE DISEASE

See cases 18, 19, 50

Definition and clinical features

Osteoporosis describes a skeletal condition in which there is an increased risk of fracture due to low bone mass and deterioration of bone microarchitecture. The World Health Organization defines osteoporosis as a bone mineral density (BMD) that is more than 2.5 standard deviations (SD) below the young average level (a so-called T score of –2.5). However, a decrease in BMD of 1 SD has also been shown to be associated with an up to threefold increased fracture risk. Thus, osteopenia is defined as T score of –1 to –2.5.

In itself, osteoporosis is asymptomatic. Symptoms arise when fractures occur. The most common sites are hip, radius and ulnar and vertebrae. All but the latter invariably lead to clinical presentation, and should therefore prompt the appropriate screening and/or treatment for osteoporosis. Vertebral fracture often goes undiagnosed. It can cause sudden onset, severe back pain, but can be mistaken for more benign mechanical back pain syndromes.

Epidemiology

Bone density begins to fall from about the age of 40 years. This loss is accelerated in women after their menopause, and also in smokers, people with low calcium intake, high alcohol consumption, low BMI and people who exercise little. In the UK, over the age of 50 years, one in two women and one in six men will fracture, and most of those will be low impact fractures, associated with osteoporosis. Incidence varies with ethnicity, for instance, it is more common in Caucasians than Afro-Caribbeans in the UK.

Osteoporosis is a well recognized complication of corticosteroid therapy. Bone loss is fastest in the early stages of treatment, and thus prevention should be considered in all patients in whom long-term corticosteroid therapy is commenced.

Differential diagnosis

Underlying abnormalities of bone metabolism should be excluded, e.g. osteomalacia and hyperparathyroidism. It may also be appropriate to screen for commonly associated comorbidities such as hyperthyroidism and diabetes mellitus.

Vertebral crush fracture can be a presentation of multiple myeloma.

Investigations

The key to diagnosis is the measurement of BMD by dual energy x-ray absorptiometry (DEXA). It may also be appropriate to perform plain x-rays to look for old vertebral insufficiency crush fractures. Absolute risk can be calculated using tools like FRAX (WHO Fracture Risk Assessment Tool).

Blood tests should include calcium, phosphate, alkaline phosphatase (ALP), vitamin D and parathyroid hormone levels.

Special points

Patients with asymptomatic vertebral crush fracture may present with a change in posture, in particular progressive kyphosis and loss of height. Again it is important to screen for osteoporosis to prevent further significant fractures. Hip fracture continues to carry a significant risk of morbidity and mortality among the elderly.

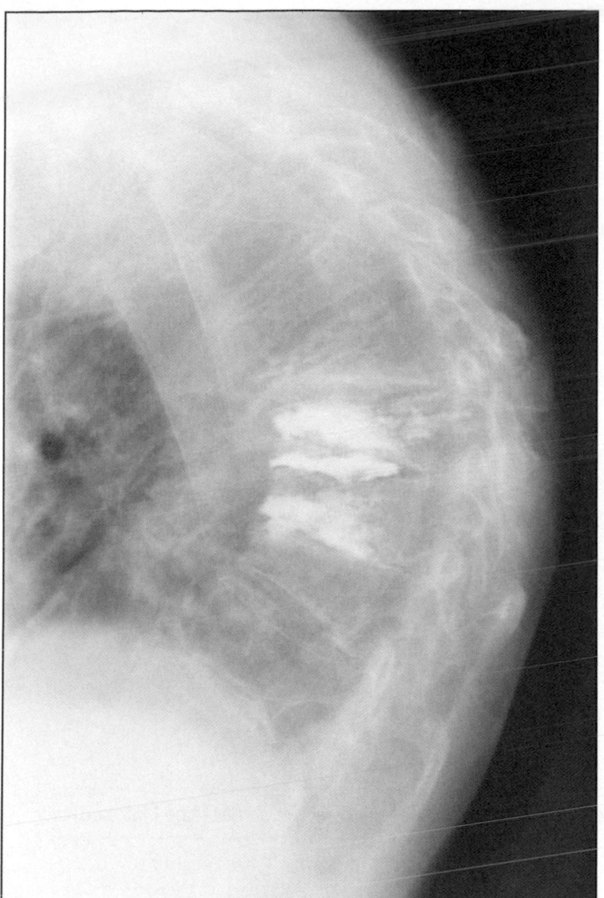

Fig. 2.43 Kyphosis with collapse of multiple mid thoracic vertebral bodies with severe calcification of the intervening discs in a patient with haemochromatosis and osteoporosis.

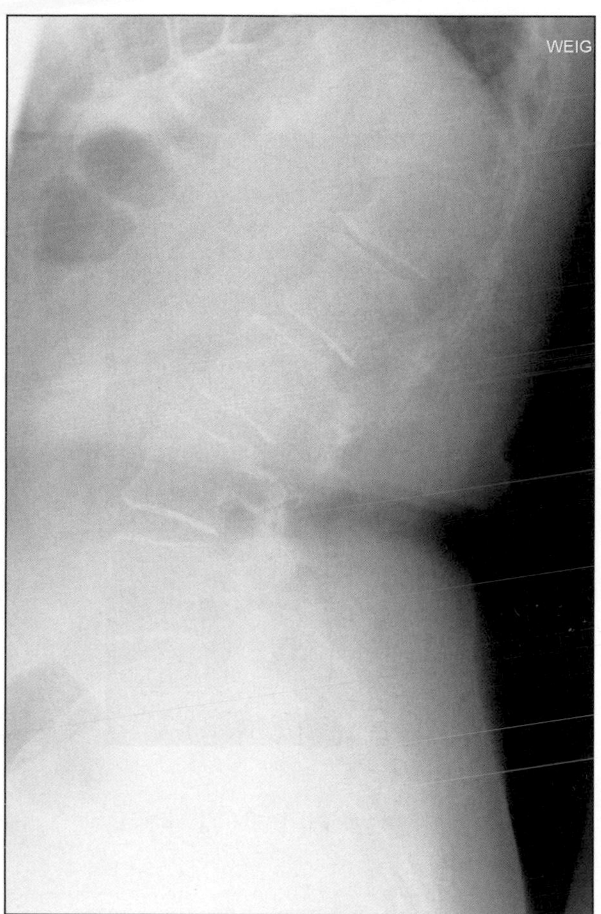

Fig. 2.44 Mild anterior wedging of T12 vertebra in a patient with postmenopausal osteoporosis and sudden onset lower thoracic back pain.

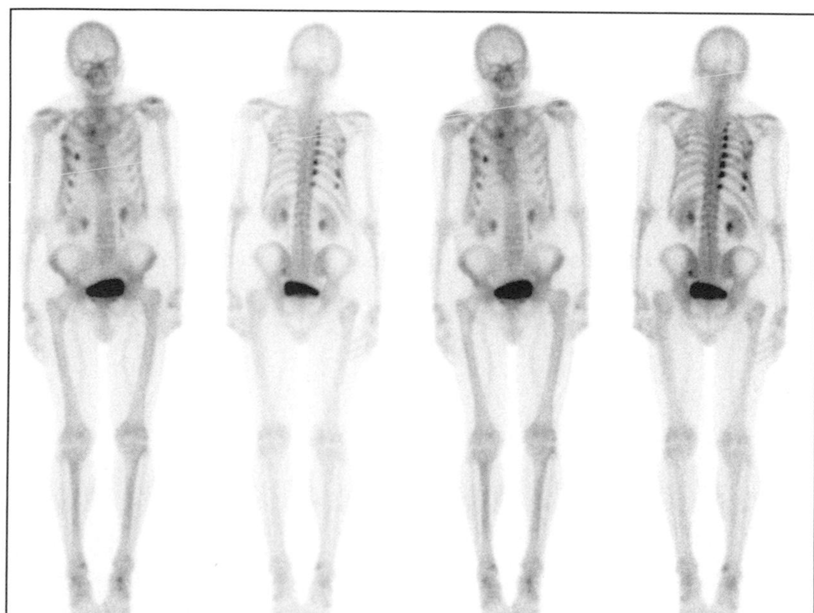

Fig. 2.45 Multiple rib fractures in a patient with long-standing osteoporosis.

a

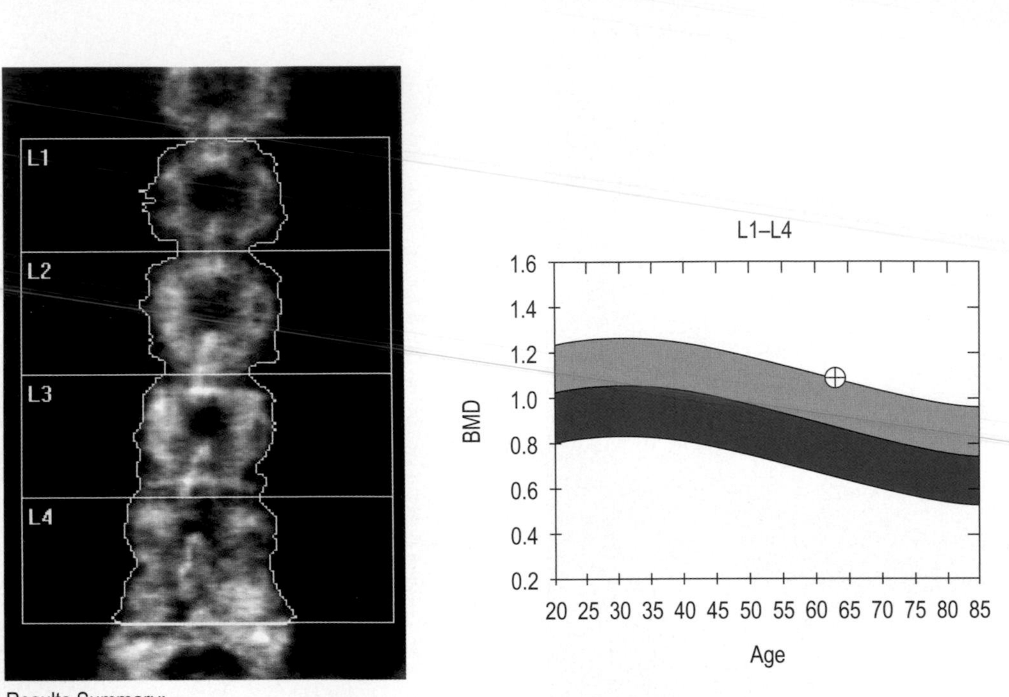

Results Summary:

Region	Area [cm^2]	BMC [(g)]	BMD [g/cm^2]	T-score	PR (Peak Reference)	Z-score	AM (Age Matched)
L1	13.24	11.70	0.884	–1.0	89	0.5	106
L2	14.87	16.01	1.077	0.4	105	2.0	126
L3	15.41	18.09	1.174	0.8	108	2.5	131
L4	19.36	22.42	1.158	0.9	109	2.6	133
Total	**62.88**	**68.23**	**1.085**	**0.3**	**104**	**2.0**	**125**

Total BMD CV 1.0%, ACF = 1.037, BCF = 1.004

Fracture Risk: Not Increased; WHO Classification: Normal

Fig. 2.46 Bone densitometry – normal bone density in spine (**2.46a**) and hip (**2.46b**).

b

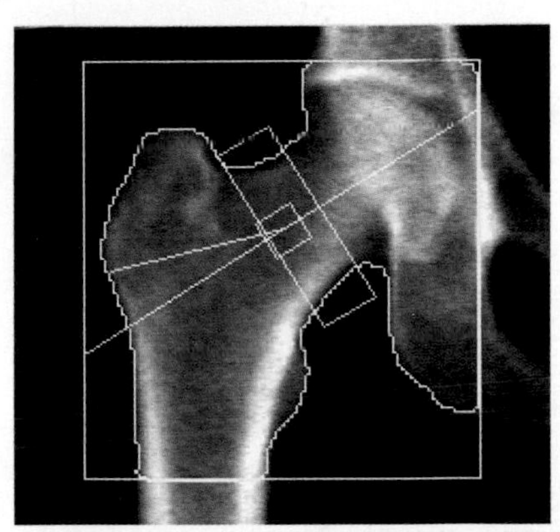

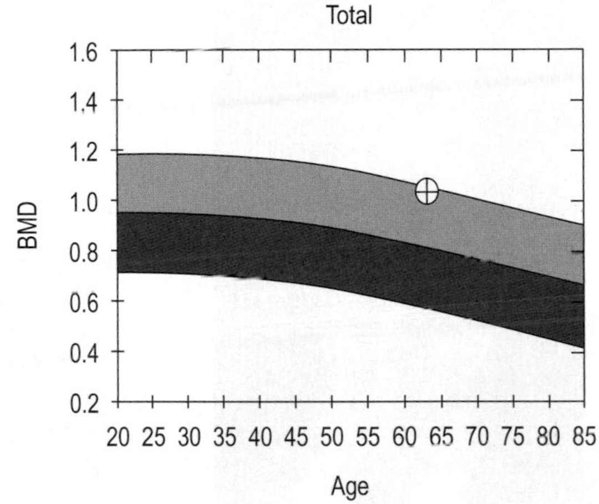

Results Summary:

Region	Area [cm^2]	BMC [(g)]	BMD [g/cm^2]	T-score	PR (Peak Reference)	Z-score	AM (Age Matched)
Neck	5.14	4.64	0.904	0.5	106	1.9	131
Troch	9.62	7.37	0.766	0.6	109	1.6	127
Inter	20.57	24.04	1.169	0.4	106	1.3	121
Total	**35.32**	**36.05**	**1.021**	**0.6**	**108**	**1.8**	**127**
Ward's	1.05	0.76	0.727	–0.6	91	2.0	144

Total BMD CV 1.0%, ACF = 1.037, BCF = 1.004

Fracture Risk: Not Increased; WHO Classification: Normal

a

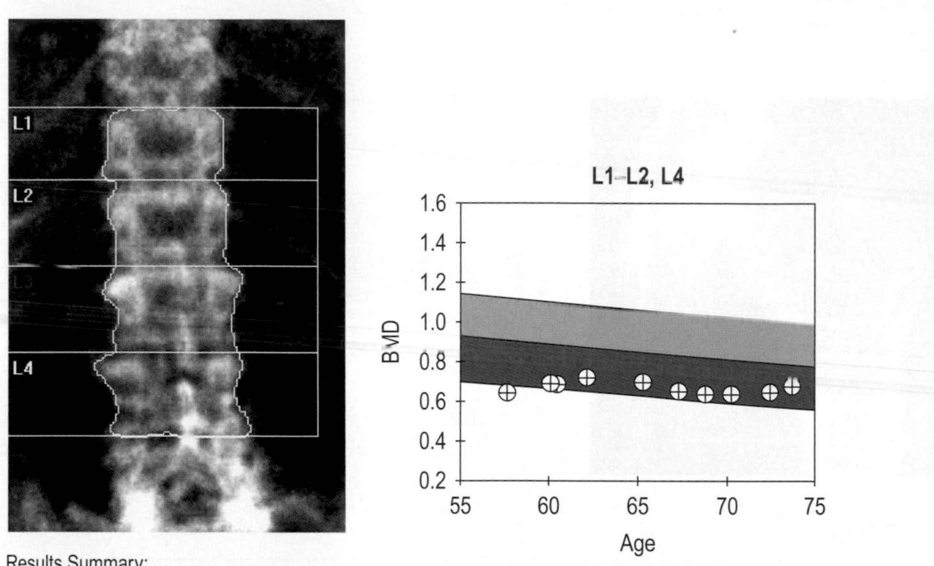

Results Summary:

Region	Area [cm²]	BMC [(g)]	BMD [g/cm²]	T-score	PR (Peak Reference)	Z-score	AM (Age Matched)
L1	11.42	7.00	0.613	–2.8	66	–0.8	88
L2	13.54	8.92	0.659	–3.4	64	–1.1	85
L4	15.77	11.65	0.738	–3.4	66	–0.9	88
Total	**40.73**	**27.57**	**0.677**	**–3.2**	**65**	**–0.9**	**87**

Total BMD CV 1.0%, ACF = 1.037, BCF = 1.004, TH = 6.373

Results History:L1–L2, L4

Scan Date	Age	BMD	T-score	BMD Change vs Baseline	BMD Change vs Previous
20.02.2012	73	0.677	–3.2	4.7%	5.0%*
18.11.2010	72	0.645	–3.5	–0.3%	1.1%
12.09.2008	70	0.638	–3.6	–1.3%	–0.2%
07.03.2007	68	0.639	–3.6	–1.1%	–1.5%
30.09.2005	67	0.649	–3.5	0.4%	–6.7%*
29.09.2003	65	0.695	–3.1	7.6%*	–3.2%*
26.07.2000	62	0.718	–2.9	11.1%*	5.3%*
15.12.1998	60	0.682	–3.2	5.4%*	–1.6%
29.07.1998	60	0.693	–3.1	7.1%*	7.1%*
30.01.1996	57	0.646	–3.5		

Fracture Risk: High; WHO Classification: Osteoporosis

* Denotes significance at 95% confidence level, LSC is 0.022326 g/cm²

Rate of change results reflect vertebral levels common to all scans.

Fig. 2.47 Bone densitometry – osteoporosis of the spine (**2.47a**) and hip (**2.47b**) in a patient with long-term steroid use. Note multiple previous results.

b

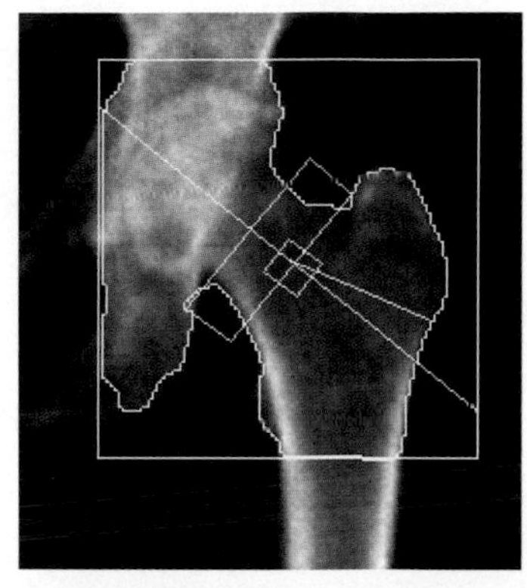

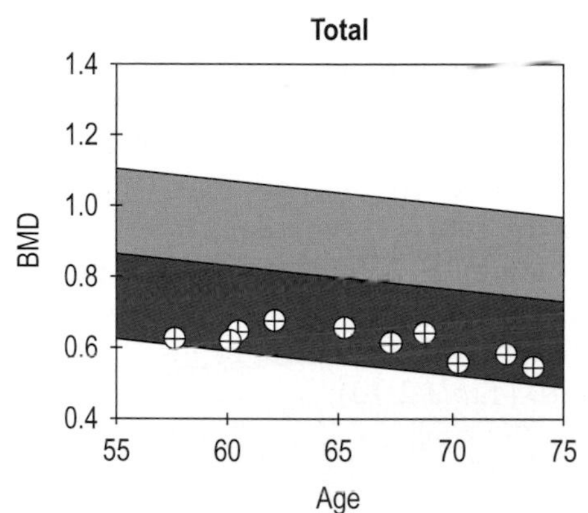

Results Summary:

Region	Area [cm^2]	BMC [(g)]	BMD [g/cm^2]	T-score	PR (Peak Reference)	Z-score	AM (Age Matched)
Neck	4.63	2.23	0.481	–3.3	57	–1.3	77
Troch	8.98	4.22	0.470	–2.3	67	–0.8	85
Inter	15.23	9.34	0.613	–3.1	56	–1.7	70
Total	**28.84**	**15.79**	**0.547**	**–3.2**	**58**	**–1.5**	**75**
Ward's	1.17	0.39	0.335	–3.4	46	–0.7	81

Total BMD CV 1.0%, ACF = 1.037, BCF = 1.004, TH = 5.069

Results History:

Scan Date	Age	BMD	T-score	BMD Change vs Baseline	BMD Change vs Previous
20.02.2012	73	0.547	–3.2	–12.5%	–5.4%*
18.11.2010	72	0.579	–3.0	–7.5%	3.5%
12.09.2008	70	0.559	–3.1	–10.6%*	–12.5%*
07.03.2007	68	0.639	–2.5	2.2%	4.9%
30.09.2005	67	0.609	–2.7	–2.6%	–7.0%*
29.09.2003	65	0.655	–2.4	4.8%*	–2.4%
26.07.2000	62	0.671	–2.2	7.3%*	4.2%
15.12.1998	60	0.644	–2.4	3.0%	4.2%
29.07.1998	60	0.618	–2.7	–1.2%	–1.2%
30.01.1996	57	0.625	–2.6		

Fracture Risk: High; WHO Classification: Osteoporosis
* Denotes significance at 95% confidence level, LSC is 0.026675 g/cm^2

10 MISCELLANEOUS RHEUMATOLOGICAL CONDITIONS

See cases 15, 20, 36, 42, 60, 78

This section is not intended to be a definitive list of rheumatological conditions, more to give the reader a feeling for the main kinds of conditions which rheumatologists come across in their daily practice. There are a few additional diagnoses which do not fit easily into the categories described thus far, and are hence grouped together here, to make up category number 10 (*Table 2.12*).

Table 2.12 Miscellaneous rheumatological conditions

Condition	Pathology	Main clinical features
Septic arthritis	Bacterial infection of a joint/ joints Common pathogens include: *Staphylococcus* spp. *Streptococcus* spp. Gonococcus	Hot, swollen joint Note, can be more than one joint Patient febrile (but not always) and unwell Increased in patients with pre-existing arthritis and in those on immunosuppressive drugs
Viral	Manifestation of systemic viral infection Common pathogens include: Parvovirus B19 Rubella Hepatitis B and C HIV	Associated with fever, and commonly rash
Sarcoidosis	Multisystem inflammatory condition characterized by the presence of non-caseating granulomas	Acute sarcoid – classic triad of ankle arthritis, erythema nodosum and bihilar lymphadenopathy
Relapsing polychondritis	Multisystem inflammatory condition characterized by the involvement of cartilage	Acute inflammation of the external ear, causing painful swelling Inner ear involvement with associated vertigo and deafness Airway involvement with collapsed bridge of nose and tracheomalacia Rash Non-erosive arthritis
Marfan's syndrome	Mutation of fibrillin gene causing defective connective tissues	Typical body habitus – tall, long arms Pectus excavatum Cardiac involvement including valve prolapse and aortic dissection and aneurysm Retinal detachment, lens dislocation Joint hypermobility Recurrent hernias Pneumothoraces
Joint hypermobility syndrome	Hypermobile, lax soft tissues	Mechanical joint pain and features of chronic pain Joint dislocation Associated with autonomic dysfunction
Complex regional pain (reflex sympathetic dystrophy, algodystrophy)	Unknown, but includes abnormal, persistent sympathetic response	Diffuse swelling and hyperalgesia/allodynia of affected limb Initially warm, then cold, pale shiny skin Often triggered by an event, e.g. disuse following trauma

REFERENCES

ACR (1999). The American College of Rheumatology nomenclature and case definitions for neuropsychiatric lupus syndromes. *Arthritis Rheum* **42**:599–608.

Aletaha D, Neogi T, Silman AJ, Funovits J, Felson DT, Bingham CO III, *et al.* (2010). Rheumatoid arthritis classification criteria: an American College of Rheumatology/European League Against Rheumatism collaborative initiative. *Arthritis Rheum* **62**:2569–2581.

Hochberg MC (1997). Updating the American College of Rheumatology revised criteria for the classification of systemic lupus erythematosus. *Arthritis Rheum* **40**:1725.

Petri M, Orbai AM, Alarcón GS, *et al.* (2012). Derivation and validation of systemic lupus international collaborating clinics classification criteria for systemic lupus erythematosus. *Arthritis Rheum* **64**:2677–2686.

Rudwaleit M, van der Heijde D, Landewé R, Listing J, Akkoc N, Brandt J, *et al.* (2009). The development of Assessment of Spondyloarthritis International Society classification criteria for axial spondyloarthritis (part II): validation and final selection. *Ann Rheum Dis* **68**:777–783.

Tan EM, Cohen AS, Fries JF, Masi AT, McShane DJ, Rothfield NF, *et al.* (1982). The 1982 revised criteria for the classification of systemic lupus erythematosus. *Arthritis Rheum* **25**:1271–1277.

Van der Linden S, Valkenburg HA, Cats A (1984). Evaluation of diagnostic criteria for ankylosing spondylitis: a proposal for modification of the New York criteria. *Arthritis Rheum* **27**:361–368.

Chapter 3

CASES

CASE 1

Six weeks following an operation a 72-year-old man was referred to the rheumatology clinic complaining of paraesthesia and numbness affecting the lateral aspect of the left leg. He had type 2 diabetes, managed with a combination of metformin and insulin. Six months previously he had been persuaded by his wife to give up smoking, and since that time, he had gained over a stone (6 kg) in weight.

On examination, he had an area of reduced sensation to light touch corresponding to the area where he experienced the paraesthesia. In addition, he had loss of pinprick sensation in a glove and stocking distribution. The rest of his neurological examination was unremarkable.

Questions

1 What is the most likely diagnosis, and what is the differential diagnosis?
2 Which investigations would you request?
3 How should the patient be managed?

CASE 2

A 52-year-old man presented with mid-lower back ache. He had a persistent ache in the right ankle where a previous x-ray had shown some ossification of the Achilles tendon. ESR, FBC, CRP and bone profile were normal.

Questions

1 Identify the main bony abnormality shown in the x-ray of his spine (**2a, 2b**).
2 In whom might this pathology be seen?
3 What complications may arise from this condition?

2a

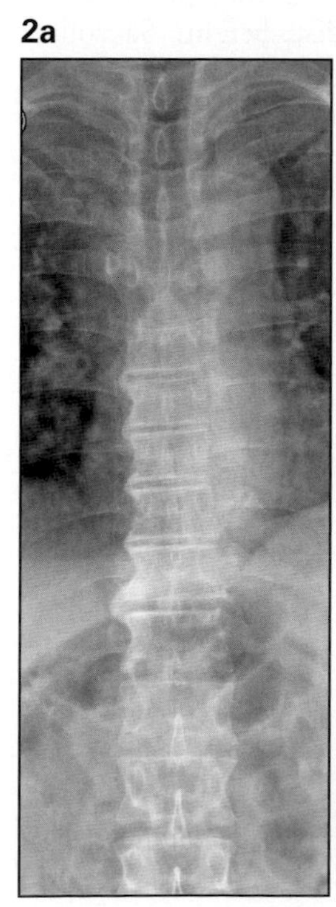

2b

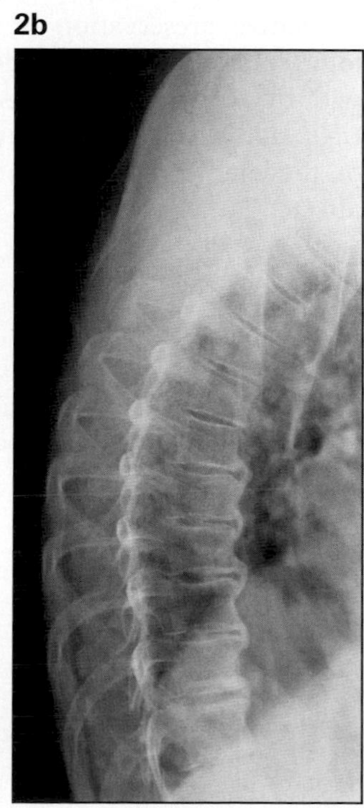

CASE 1

Answers

1 Meralgia paraesthetica is the most likely diagnosis – in view of recent surgery, and weight gain, both risk factors, in combination with the common peripheral neuropathy of diabetes. The differential diagnosis includes diabetic amyotrophy, lumbar plexopathy and L2 radiculopathy.
2 HbA1c test and nerve conduction studies should be performed.
3 Management is generally conservative with lifestyle advice such as weight loss and wearing loose clothes. Drugs which are effective for neuropathic pain such as amitriptyline and gabapentin can be used, and occasionally if very severe, patients may opt for surgical release.

Outcome

His nerve conduction studies showed a mild axonal neuropathy, consistent with his diabetes. The fact that he required insulin in addition to metformin would imply that his disease control had been poor, increasing his risk of the diabetic complications. In addition, there was no evidence of L2 radiculopathy on the EMG. Direct studies of the lateral cutaneous nerve of the thigh can be done, but are not usually necessary.

CASE 2

Answers

1 The x-ray shows diffuse idiopathic skeletal hyperostosis (DISH), also known as Forestier's disease – note the ossification of the anterior longitudinal ligament along the thoracic spine (like candle wax dripping along the spine). There is relative preservation of disc height. Sacroiliac joint erosion, sclerosis or fusion is not associated with this condition. The disease usually affects the right side of the spine because of aortic pulsations on the left. Thoracic vertebrae are most commonly affected.
2 DISH usually affects patients over age 50 years. It is more frequent in patients with type 2 diabetes, hyperlipidaemia and/or hyperuricaemia. Only 8% of white patients with DISH will be HLA-B27 positive.
3 Complications are rare; however, the condition may cause dysphagia when the flowing spinal cervical hyperostosis encroaches on the pharynx and oesophagus. Thoracic lesions may compress the bronchi or the inferior venae cavae. Nerve root compression may also occur.

CASE 3

A 22-year-old Caucasian woman had received an insect bite on her lower leg which developed into an ulcer which did not seem to heal. She was also noted to have had two spontaneous abortions, was complaining of some polyarthralgia in her hands and feet and on testing had a low platelet count of 70 × 10^9/l. The patient was referred to the rheumatology department where the history was confirmed and a complex, social history of soft drug dependency – 'marijuana seems to ease the pain' – was noted. There was nothing else of relevance in her previous history and on examination a large ulcer just above the lateral malleolus was noted (**3a**, **3b**). Although her pulse was normal at 80 bpm her blood pressure was increased at 150/100 mmHg but urinalysis was normal. Renal and liver function tests were normal but her glomerular filtration rate was a little reduced at 60 ml/min. Her low platelet count was confirmed (down to 30 × 10^9/l).

Over the next year her ulcer failed to heal and her high blood pressure proved difficult to control in spite of using a combination of three antihypertensives. Approximately 14 months after she was seen in the rheumatology clinic she suffered a cerebrovascular accident, affecting her left side.

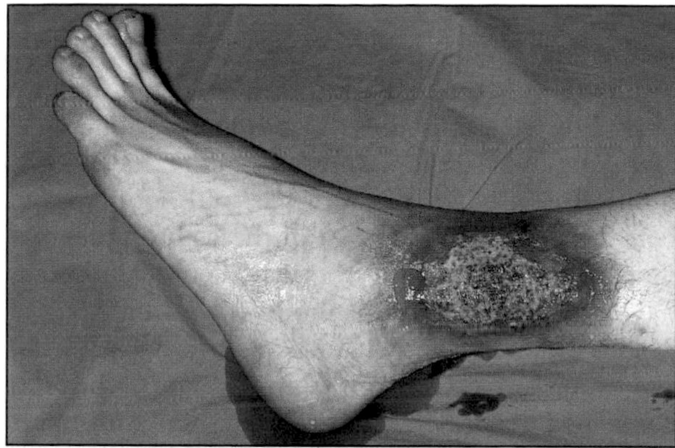

3a

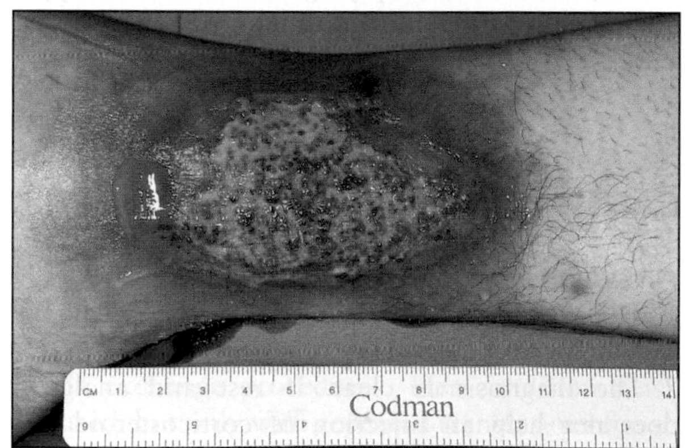

3b

Questions

1 What set of blood tests need to be done to clinch the diagnosis?
2 What possible link might explain the leg ulcer with the diagnosis?
3 Why is this patient hypertensive?
4 What two possible causes of her stroke can you think of?
5 What key investigation is needed, prior to starting her on treatment?

CASE 4

A 50-year-old slim and fit woman presented with a 6-month history of increasing pain in the left hip. When asked to be more specific, she pointed to the lateral hip. It was painful to lie on the left side at night and walking and stairs were also painful. Running was impossible, which for her was a problem as she ran to keep fit. She was otherwise well and recalled no injury. On examination it was painful to adduct the flexed hip. The hip joint showed a normal range of movement. She was tender over the greater trochanter. The lumbar spine moved freely and there was no scoliosis. X-ray of the pelvis was normal.

Questions

1 What is the most likely diagnosis?
2 How would you treat the patient?
3 What is the differential diagnosis of lateral hip pain?
4 If the pain persists what is the best method for investigating the patient?

CASE 5

Answers

1 Initial therapy should be with high dose NSAIDs, but if the arthritis doesn't resolve swiftly, then oral steroids should be considered in the short term and DMARD therapy, typically with sulphasalazine, if necessary. Eradication of the streptococcal infection with penicillin is generally advocated, and tonsillectomy may be considered in some recalcitrant cases, though is more difficult in late adolescence/adulthood than in younger children.

2 When compared to the classic HLA-B27-associated reactive arthritis secondary to gastrointestinal or genitourinary infections, PSRA more commonly involves joints of the upper limb and is generally associated with a better outcome.

CASE 6

Answers

1 The patient has systemic lupus erythematosus (SLE) with active glomerulonephritis. However, a list of her immediate problems includes haemolytic anaemia, thrombocytopenia, biopsy-proven microangiopathy in small renal vessels, renal failure and malignant hypertension with seizures. These features are strong indicators for autoimmune-associated thrombotic thrombocytopenic purpura (TTP).

In recent years there have been over 100 case reports of TTP-like syndromes in lupus patients, and partial TTP-like syndromes are relatively common in SLE. Autopsy studies suggest that microangiopathy is more common in lupus than is generally appreciated clinically and some suggest that the nephropathy of the anti-phospholipid syndrome, with small vessel occlusions, could be considered a partial variant of TTP. Classic TTP arises from a genetic polymorphism in the Von Willebrand-cleaving ADAMTS-13 protease. Autoimmune-associated TTP-like syndromes appear to be antibody-mediated, affecting the same pathway, which results in the accumulation of Von Willebrand factor multimers and associated vasculopathy.

This patient's problems are also suggestive of the catastrophic anti-phospholipid syndrome (CAPS). First described by Asherson in 1992, CAPS is characterized by rapid onset of multiorgan failure due to small vessel thrombi in the context of anti-phospholipid antibodies. Data from the International CAPS registry confirm that 70% of CAPS patients have renal involvement, 60% may have cerebral involvement, 68% have thrombocytopenia and 26% have evidence for haemolysis. It has recently been appreciated that CAPS and TTP may exist along a continuum of microangiopathic syndromes with overlapping features, which also include haemolytic uraemic syndrome, preeclampsia and scleroderma renal crisis.

2 Regardless of diagnosis, the treatment for autoimmune TTP and CAPS is identical, including prompt institution of plasma exchange, aggressive steroids, heparin, and in some cases additional immunosuppression (although this remains more controversial). Early and aggressive treatment seems to have a significant impact on the otherwise poor prognosis.

CASE 7

A 73-year-old man with chronic renal impairment presented with a predominantly small joint arthritis. His hands and feet are shown (7**a**, 7**b**) together with the x-rays (7**c**, 7**d**).

Questions

1 Describe the patent's hands and feet.
2 Describe the x-ray findings.
3 What is the diagnosis?
4 How should the patient be managed?

7a

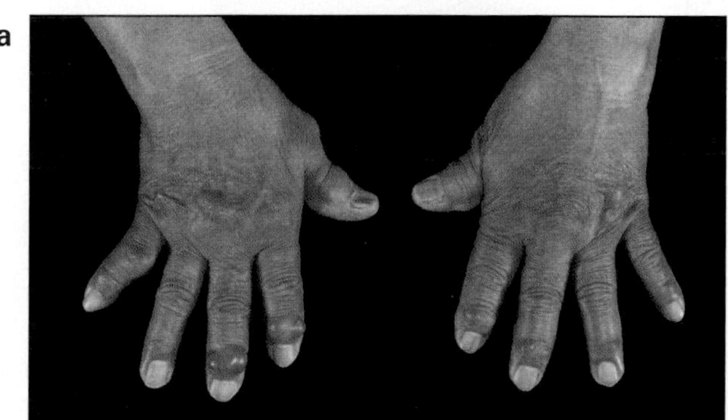

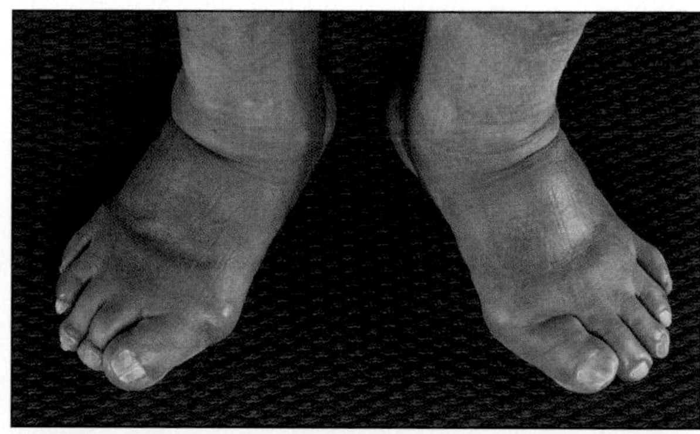

7b

7c

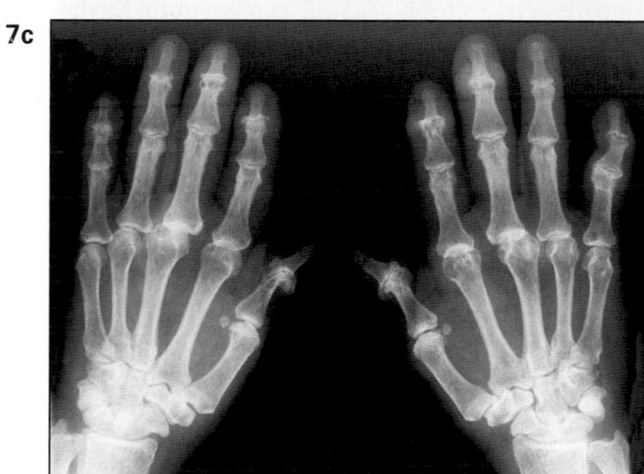

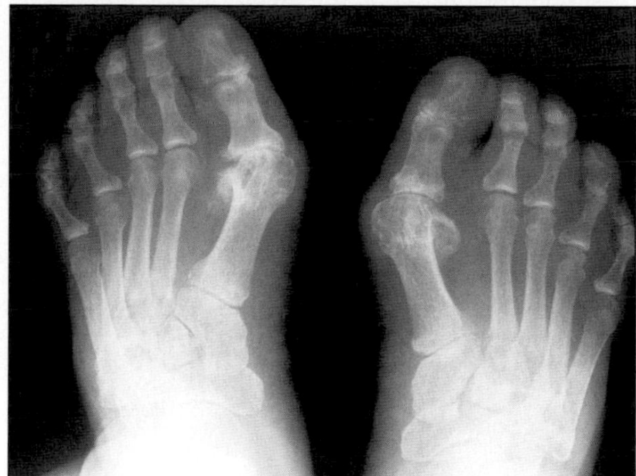

7d

CASE 8

A 63-year-old woman presented with a 2-day history of low grade fever, myalgia, fatigue and a dull aching bitemporal headache associated with right sided scalp tenderness. Her past medical history included: myopia, surgical correction of left strabismus 16 years ago and infrequent right sided migraine headaches usually preceded by an aura.

On examination her visual acuity was 6/6 in the right eye and 6/24 in the left correcting to 6/6 with spectacles. Ocular pressures, visual fields and optic discs were normal. The right temporal artery was tender with reduced pulsatility and mild erythema of the surrounding scalp. Her temperature was 38.8°C. Examination of the chest, abdomen, CNS and joints revealed no abnormalities.

Questions

1 What is the most likely diagnosis?
2 What main investigations should be included in the diagnostic workup?
3 What should initial management be?

CASE 7

Answers

1 He has yellow-coloured subcutaneous deposits overlying his distal interphalangeal (DIP) joints and the interphalangeal (IP) joints of both thumbs, with overlying tight, shiny skin. He has evidence of a destructive arthritis predominantly affecting the same joints. The picture of his feet shows peripheral oedema, suggesting ongoing problems with fluid balance, bilateral hallux valgus and swelling of the right fourth toe.

2 The x-rays of his hands show soft tissue swelling around the DIPs. He has widespread erosions, which are round/oval in shape and have sclerotic margins. The erosions are associated with overhanging margins of bone, particularly around the IP joints of both thumbs. He has lost joint space with sclerotic joint margins, a sign of coexisting osteoarthritis and of long-standing disease. The x-rays of his feet show erosions predominantly affecting the first metatarsophalangeal joints, with significant bony outgrowth.

3 Chronic tophaceous gout. Serum uric acid levels were 550 μmol/l, consistent with his renal impairment.

4 First line treatment should be with allopurinol, with colchicine cover (NSAIDs are avoided in this case because of renal impairment). Typically, allopurinol should be started at 100 mg/day, and titrated up depending upon serum uric acid. Adequate therapy can lead to resolution, or at least improvement, of tophi, as well as preventing further acute gouty attacks.

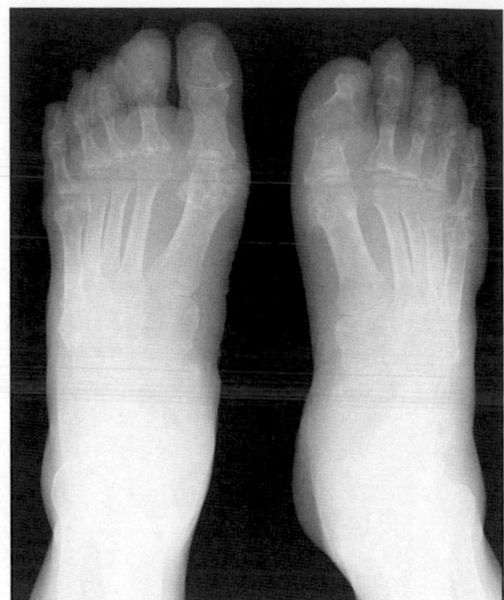

7e

Discussion

While gout most commonly causes acute, resolving attacks of arthritis, tophaceous gout is associated with a destructive, chronic arthropathy. **Figure 7e** shows an x-ray of another patient with chronic tophaceous gout. Note the absence of bone/joint around the IP joint of the right great toe. This is due to complete destruction by a large gouty tophus.

CASE 8

Answers

1 The history and clinical findings strongly suggest a diagnosis of giant cell arteritis (GCA).

2 Further investigations should include ESR, CRP, platelet count, haemoglobin and temporal artery biopsy. An ESR of 50 mm/h or greater is 86.5% sensitive and 47.7% specific in predicting positive biopsy results. The ESR is normal in 2–8% of patients with biopsy-proven GCA. Both ESR and CRP are useful for monitoring treatment response. The CRP changes more rapidly in response to inflammatory activity and is more useful in monitoring older patients or those who have other haematological conditions such as monoclonal gammopathies.

A temporal artery biopsy will distinguish between GCA and other vasculitides which may rarely involve the temporal artery. The diagnostic yield is greater if at least 2 cm of artery is biopsied. Bilateral biopsy only improves the yield in 3% of cases.

3 In the absence of visual, CNS or other complications, initial management should be with oral prednisolone. Most clinicians start with 40 mg/day or 0.75–1 mg/kg to a maximum of 60 mg/day and taper once there is normalization of both symptoms and inflammatory markers. Alternate day dosing is less effective in producing remission. Proton pump inhibitors for gastroprotection, and bone protectants such as a bisphosphonate should be added. Dietary counselling regarding adequate calcium and vitamin D intake should be offered.

CASE 9

A woman aged 45 years presented to her family practitioner complaining of dryness of the eyes and mouth. She had a previous history of sarcoidosis in her mid-twenties and was complaining of some low grade polyarthralgia. She was therefore referred by her primary care physician to the local rheumatology unit.

As well as the above history, she confirmed that the sarcoidosis had principally involved her chest and her old notes confirmed she had had bihilar lymphadenopathy which had been treated for a short period with corticosteroids, with which she had become asymptomatic and her chest x-ray returned to normal.

The patient confirmed that her eyes, as well as being dry, were itchy, irritable and photosensitive. Dryness of the mouth was particularly troublesome at night. She was not having trouble with any swelling of her peripheral joints though she confirmed that they did ache intermittently throughout the day.

On taking a family history, she mentioned that she had had four children and that two of them had had some kind of heart problem when they were born and that one of them had had a transient skin rash. Both children were fitted with pacemakers for some years but now in their early teens they seemed to be doing very well. She was asked to bring a photograph (9) of one of these two children to the next clinic appointment.

On examination an absence of the salivary pool beneath the tongue was evident and the tongue looked dry. There was no sign of synovitis. Examination of her cardiovascular system, respiratory system, abdomen and CNS was normal.

Questions

1 Could the dryness of the eyes and mouth be due to sarcoidosis and if so, what test(s) would you do to prove the diagnosis?
2 Could the dryness of the eyes and mouth be due to Sjögren's syndrome – what test(s) would you do to confirm the diagnosis?
3 What serological abnormalities are likely to be linked to the appearances that are shown in the photograph?
4 What is the most likely outcome of the clinical features shown in the photograph?
5 What other internal organ is most strongly associated with the clinical feature shown in the picture and how is it treated?

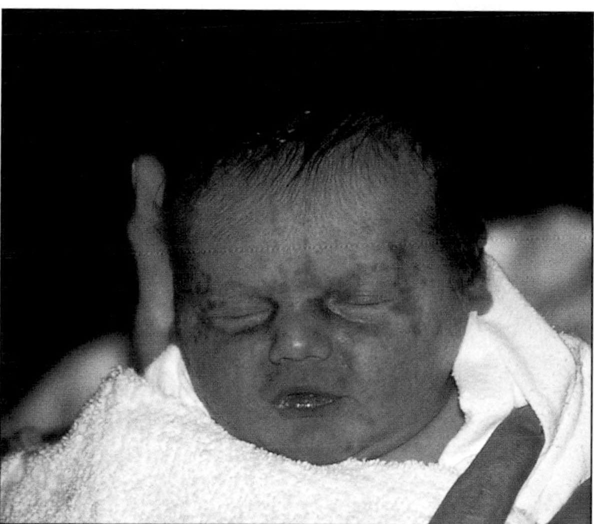

9

CASE 12

Answers

1 The films show Charcot joint.

2 To investigate the neuropathy she needs neurophysiology with nerve conduction studies and EMG. She also requires genetic testing.

3 The patient has Charcot–Marie–Tooth (CMT) syndrome. She needs to consider genetic screening for family members.

Discussion

There are two types of CMT which can present in adulthood. CMT type 1 is due to a mutation in the peripheral myelin protein-22 gene, which results in demyelination, and hence slowing of nerve conduction. CMT type 2 results in direct axonal death. Patients usually present by the age of 20 years, but some mutations lead to milder clinical pictures, and hence present later.

The neuropathy affects both sensory and motor fibres, and accordingly causes loss of sensation in addition to muscle bulk loss and weakness. Classically, muscle loss starts distally, producing 'inverted champagne bottle legs'. In addition to weakness, patients present complaining of musculoskeletal and neuropathic pain, as in this case.

Management includes physiotherapy, orthotics and occasionally surgery. Genetic counselling is also crucial for those considering having children.

CASE 13

Answers

1 This patient meets criteria for primary anti-phospholipid syndrome and is at high risk for recurrent thrombosis.

2 Antiplatelet therapy appears to be effective in preventing recurrent strokes in these and other stroke-prone patients, and should certainly be a part of the management in this case. However, the patient's young age and severe history support consideration of adding additional treatment, perhaps a judicious combination of antiplatelet and moderate dose coumarin or antithrombin treatments. There is no evidence based literature to support immune suppression for the anti-phospholipid syndrome, but it is of interest that a recurrent stroke occurred 6 months after rituximab therapy, possibly consistent with the reconstitution of the B cell population. Empiric use of such treatments is increasing, and it can be hoped that further information about the results of such use will become available.

This patient's list of symptoms suggests the possibility that she will evolve to the diagnosis of systemic lupus, but at the present time most of her most concrete features are localized to the haematological system. Lupus-like features are common in patients with anti-phospholipid syndrome which, like other partial lupus syndromes, could be considered a forme fruste of systemic autoimmunity.

CASE 14

A 45-year-old keen badminton player who kept fit at the gym presented with a 4-month history of medial elbow pain. The pain was made worse by carrying heavy files and by lifting weights. He was otherwise fit and well. There was localized tenderness over the medial epicondyle and this was made worse by flexing the wrist against resistance with the arm straight.

Questions

1 What is the diagnosis?
2 How would you treat this patient?
3 What are other common causes of pain around the elbow?

CASE 15

A 35-year-old woman was referred to the chest physicians with a 1-month history of progressive shortness of breath on exertion. She had been diagnosed with systemic lupus erythematosus (SLE) 4 years previously when she presented with malar rash, oral ulcers, photosensitivity and ANA titre 1:1,280. Her disease had been uncomplicated over the years, and she had been taking hydroxychloroquine 400 mg daily for fatigue and arthralgia.

On examination, she was afebrile, her chest was clear, and cardiac examination was normal. Nodular lesions were noted on her legs (**15a**) and curious papular lesions on her upper back (**15b**).

Blood investigations revealed Hb of 11.8 g/dl and ESR 46 mm/h; d-dimers were negative and tests for anti-phospholipid antibodies were negative; blood cultures revealed no growth of organisms after 5 days.

A chest x-ray showed bilateral hilar lymphadenopathy.

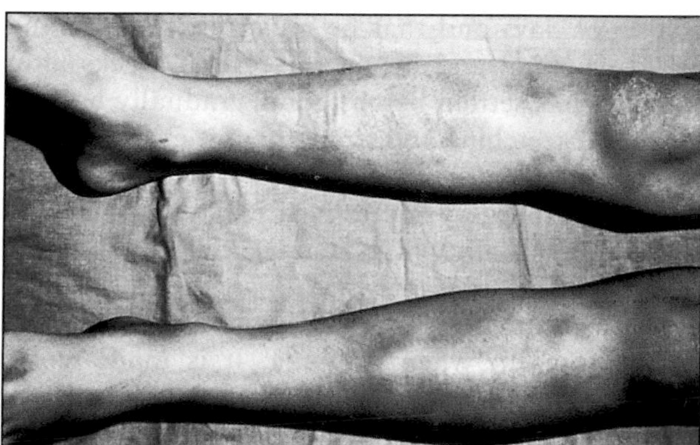

15a

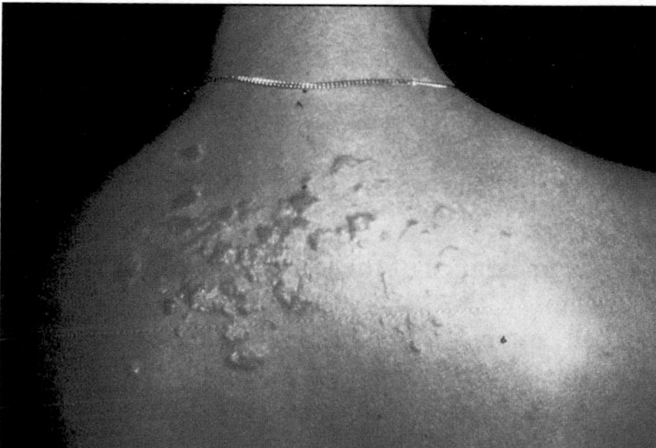

15b

Questions

1 Identify the lesions on her legs and back.
2 List three important differential diagnoses.
3 What further investigations may be helpful in reaching a diagnosis?

CASE 19

Answers

1 The findings are compatible with osteoporosis at the hip (T score –2.5 overall, worst at Ward's triangle) and in the spine (T score –3.7).

2 She should be screened for any underlying metabolic cause which might contribute to the loss of bone density. This should include a full medical history and examination to establish whether there are untreated inflammatory diseases. Review of medication may also provide useful information, for instance regarding steroid or antiepileptic medication use. Serum should be tested for vitamin D and parathyroid hormone levels. It may also be useful to get a plain x-ray of the thoracic and lumbar spine to look for asymptomatic crush fractures. This is also useful in terms of having baseline imaging which can then be used to assess disease progression. Finally, it is unusual for bone mineral density to fall in a patient taking regular bisphosphonates, and it therefore may be appropriate to address the issue of adherence. Compliance with bisphosphonate treatment should lead to a fall in bone turnover markers such as collagen type 1 telopeptide. A lack of suppression would therefore suggest poor adherence to treatment.

3 Assuming that there is no underlying cause identified from the above investigations, it is necessary to change treatment. Strontium ranelate would be a sensible next choice, and if this is not tolerated, IV pamidronate could be used. Further fractures would be an indication for teriparatide.

4 Response to treatment should be assessed by repeat bone densitometry every 2–3 years, and screening for new vertebral crush fractures with plain films.

5 Symptoms and x-ray findings are compatible with an acute vertebral crush fracture of L5.

6 A myeloma screen should be done to exclude this as the cause of the collapse. In terms of management, in the short term these patients require a significant amount of analgesia, sometimes including opiates. In addition, IV pamidronate or subcutaneous salmon calcitonin can also be used. Longer term, treatment with teriparatide would be indicated.

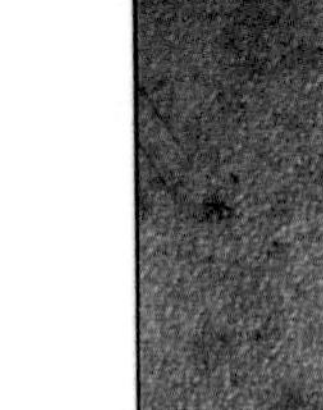

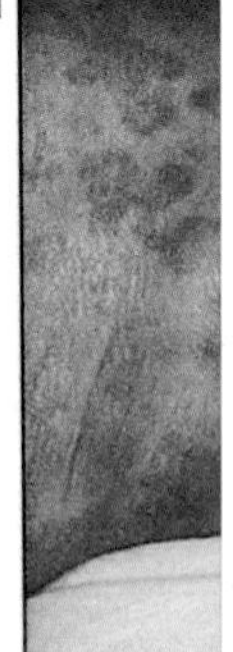

CASE 20

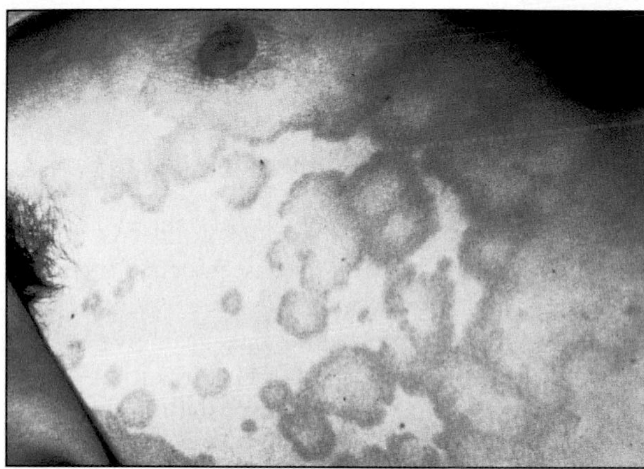

20

An 8-year-old Turkish girl presented to the emergency department with a 3-day history of an erythematous non-pruritic rash on the chest (**20**) and back associated with fever, malaise and pain in the ankles. The ankle pains had resolved after 18 hours, but then she noticed pain in the right wrist followed by painful swelling of the left knee.

She had been previously fit and well, but 2 weeks prior to the onset of her rash and joint pains, she had complained of a sore throat that seemed to have improved after 2 days of home therapy with aspirin gargles and antiseptic lozenges.

Examination findings were as follows. Temperature 38.3°C; BP 96/54 mmHg; pulse 96/min, regular; respiratory rate 20/min; tonsils enlarged, mild pharyngeal injection; chest clear; grade 1/VI systolic murmur at the lower left sternal edge; right wrist warm, mildly swollen and tender. Abdomen and CNS showed no abnormalities.

There was no rash visible on the face, hands or feet.

Laboratory results were as follows: Hb 12.9 g/dl, WBC 12.6 × 10^9/l with 76% neutrophils, 14% lymphocytes, 2% eosinophils, 6% reactive lymphocytes, 2% monocytes, platelets 430 × 10^9/l, ESR 78 mm/h, CRP 10.2 mg/l, ANA negative, RF negative, ASO titre 360 Todd units, viral serology negative; knee aspirate – no organisms on Gram stain, no crystals seen.

Questions

1 Identify the rash and make the diagnosis.
2 How should the patient be managed?

CASE 21

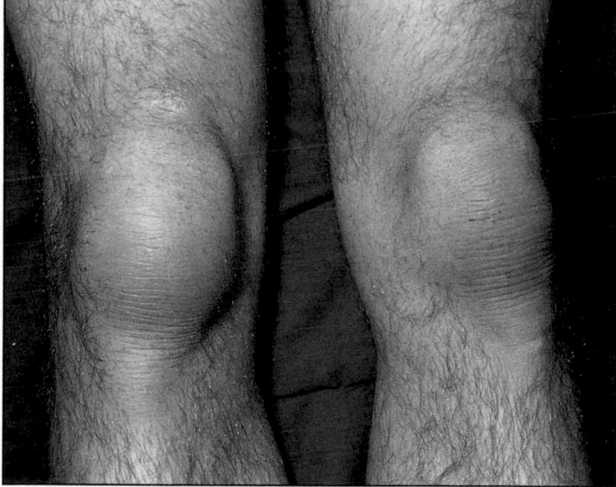

21

This male patient had recently spent 5 days laying laminate flooring in his house. By day 3, he noticed pain, swelling and tenderness over the knee caps (**21**) with mild discomfort on flexing the knees. He remained otherwise well in himself.

Questions

1 What is the most likely cause of the patient's painful knees?
2 What other conditions may give rise to this complaint?
3 What diagnostic tests are indicated?
4 What intervention would you recommend for this patient?

CASE 20

Answers

1 Erythema marginatum. The patient has arthritis and erythema marginatum which are two of the five revised major Jones criteria needed to make a diagnosis of rheumatic fever. The presence of fever and raised inflammatory markers fulfil two minor criteria, and in addition she has evidence of recent pharyngeal infection with group A streptococci.

A rapid streptococcal antigen test can give a quick indication of the presence of infection with group A streptococci. Throat cultures are usually negative at the time of onset of symptoms of rheumatic fever; however, streptococcal antibody levels usually peak at this time. The ASO titre was only moderately raised in this patient. Values of 200–300 Todd units are not uncommonly seen in healthy schoolchildren and carriers of group A streptococci. Serial ASO titres checked 2 weeks apart may reveal progressive rise in ASO titre followed by a fall as the disease resolves. Up to 20% of group A streptococci will not produce ASO, hence other streptococcal antibody tests may be employed to increase the sensitivity of the results. These additional tests include: the anti-DNAase B test which detects antibodies against the deoxyribonuclease B enzyme produced by most group A streptococci; antistreptokinase and antihyaluronidase.

2 The patient should be further evaluated by way of ECG and echocardiogram for the presence of carditis. Medical management includes: bed rest, aspirin (70 mg/kg/day in divided doses) aiming to keep aspirin blood levels at 20–25 mg/dl; and streptococcal eradication with oral penicillin V for 10 days, or a single dose of IM benzathine penicillin (0.6–1.2 million units).

Aspirin usually causes resolution of arthritis within 24–36 hours but treatment should be continued until inflammatory markers normalize. This may take up to 6 weeks.

There are WHO guidelines for penicillin prophylaxis for patients with rheumatic fever. Duration of treatment varies depending on the presence of rheumatic carditis. This patient will require penicillin prophylaxis until the age of 21 years.

CASE 21

Answers

1 The pain is probably due to prepatellar bursitis (bilateral) – also known as housemaid's knee. It has been caused in this case by recurrent minor trauma due to excessive kneeling.

2 Other conditions might be a septic or pyogenic process, inflammatory diseases such as rheumatoid arthritis or crystal deposition diseases.

3 The diagnosis is usually made based on the history and clinical findings. If septic bursitis is suspected, then the bursa should be aspirated and fluid samples sent for microbiological analysis. Fluid microscopy may also reveal other causes of the prepatellar bursitis including monosodium urate crystals seen in gout.

4 Recommended treatment is simple analgesics and/or NSAIDs; there should be a short period of rest followed by physical therapy, patient education, avoidance of excessive kneeling and use of knee pads.

CASE 22

A 66-year-old man was referred to the orthopaedic clinic with right hip and groin pain. Twelve years earlier he had had a left total hip replacement following a diagnosis of osteoarthritis. X-rays of his hips revealed mild osteoarthritis on the right, and no problems with the replacement on the left. On further questioning he admitted to abdominal pain, malaise and an unspecified amount of weight loss. Examination revealed pain-free movements of both hips with generalized abdominal tenderness. His CRP was 30.2 mg/l, but all other blood tests including FBC and renal liver function tests were normal. An ultrasound of his abdomen revealed an infrarenal abdominal aortic aneurysm measuring 4.1 cm in diameter. This was confirmed on a CT abdomen which also showed surrounding inflammatory change with retroperitoneal lymphadenopathy.

The patient was referred to rheumatology for advice about definitive diagnosis and management.

Questions

1 What other important information is required from the history?
2 What imaging should be done?
3 What is the differential diagnosis?

CASE 23

A 23-year-old woman of Afro-Caribbean origin presented with swelling of both legs to mid calf, increasing fatigue and hair loss. She had also been troubled by some intermittent swelling of her joints with early morning stiffness lasting over an hour. There was little of relevance in her previous medical history and no family history of note. She had been prescribed some furosemide by her primary care physician which had not made much difference.

On examination she had bilateral pitting oedema to mid calf with diffuse alopecia. Her blood pressure was 150/100 mmHg and significant axillary lymphadenopathy was noted. There were no other clinical findings.

Initial investigations showed Hb to be 10.2 g/dl with normal iron indices, normal WBC and normal platelet count. The urea and creatinine were just above the upper limit of normal but her liver function tests were within the normal limits. Her ANA was raised to 1:640 diffuse pattern with antibodies to dsDNA detectable by the *Crithidia* method. Urine analysis revealed proteinuria 3+ with red cell casts more than 20 per high power field noted.

Over the next 3 months she was treated with oral prednisolone and azathioprine, which initially seemed to be helpful. Her urea and creatinine returned to normal but her hypertension remained difficult to control and she had persistent heavy proteinuria. In addition, she was becoming increasingly concerned about her hair loss (**23**).

Questions

1 What percentage of patients with systemic lupus erythematosus suffer from either significant renal disease or from alopecia?
2 Antibodies to dsDNA are often associated with renal lupus; what other autoantibodies are linked to subsets of lupus's clinical features?
3 What clinical feature is shown in the figure and what are the treatment options?
4 Given that the combination of prednisolone and azathioprine seems to have failed to control this patient's renal disease, what other options are now available?

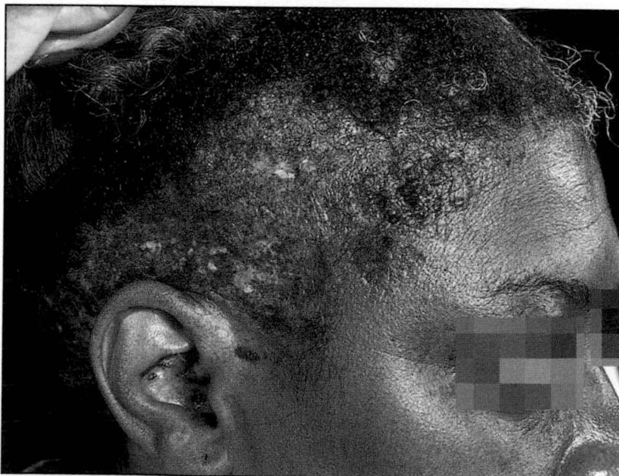

23

CASE 22

ANSWERS

1 Are there any features of a giant cell arteritis (GCA)? Ask about temporal headaches and tenderness, jaw claudication and visual disturbance. Are there features of polymyalgia rheumatica (PMR). In this case, the patient described malaise, but no other features of GCA or PMR.

2 The key question in this patient with an inflammatory aortitis is whether the changes are confined to the abdominal aorta, or are more generalized. The choice is between angiography, CT, MRI or CT with FDG-PET.

3 The differential diagnosis here is between a localized plaque associated abdominal aortic aneurysm, or a more generalized large vessel vasculitis. The significant retroperitoneal fibrosis suggests an inflammatory pathology.

Outcome

In this case, an FDG-PET/CT was done (22) and shows increased FDG activity in the thoracic and abdominal aorta, and the axillary, subclavian and brachiocephalic vessels, compatible with a large vessel vasculitis. This patient is the wrong age and sex for Takayasu's disease, and had none of the associated clinical features. He had no clinical features of GCA, and retroperitoneal fibrosis is not a common association with this condition. The diagnosis in this case is chronic periaortitis (CP). CP is an idiopathic fibroinflammatory condition in which large vessel vasculitis (predominantly aortitis) is associated with retroperitoneal fibrosis. The treatment is immunosuppression with corticosteroids (prednisolone 1 mg/kg), tapered in a similar way to patients with GCA. Steroid-sparing agents such as methotrexate or azathioprine may be needed. In this case, the patient responded rapidly to oral steroids, with improvement in symptoms and normalization of his CRP. Over 3 months, the size of his abdominal aortic aneurysm had reduced to 3.7 cm. Follow-up PET/CT was planned for 6 months to assess response.

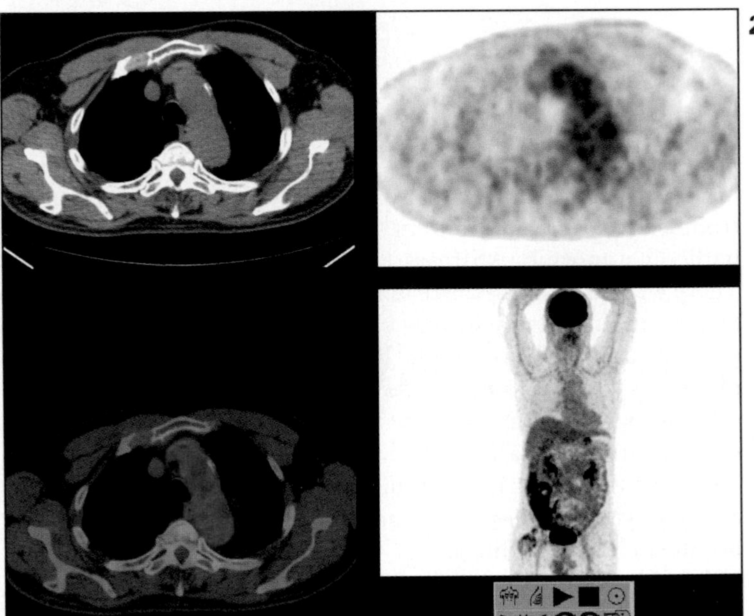

22

CASE 23

ANSWERS

1 Significant renal disease is found in 30–40% of lupus patients. Transient local or diffuse alopecia has been reported in approximately 20–35% of most series, though scarring alopecia is much less common, being seen in 5% or fewer.

2 Anti-Ro is linked with photosensitivity and neonatal lupus; anti-La with Sjögren's syndrome; and anti-phospholipid antibodies with recurrent thromboses and miscarriages.

3 The treatment of scarring alopecia shown in the figure is profoundly unsatisfactory. Rarely, increasing the systemic immunosuppression may be helpful and occasionally intralesional steroids may be of some value, but very often the preferred option is to use a wig.

4 Options would include cyclophosphamide, mycophenolate or rituximab.

CASE 24

A 32-year-old man presented with a sudden onset of severe pain and stiffness of the neck. He had pain at the base of the neck and in the left medial shoulder blade. He worked at a computer all day under great stress as a securities trader. There was no injury. He was barely able to move the neck and held it to one side. Shoulder movement was normal. He did not have arm pain.

Questions

1 What is the differential diagnosis of this patient's pain?
2 How would you treat the patient?
3 If the pain did not settle in 3 weeks, what investigation would you do?

CASE 25

A 33-year-old Caucasian woman presented with a 2-year history of progressive polyarticular arthritis involving bilateral fingers, knees, feet and shoulders. Her previous treatment had been with a combination of narcotics and low dose methotrexate (7.5 mg/week). Review of systems was notable for 2 hours of morning stiffness, active pain, tenderness and swelling in the hands and feet, which made it difficult for her to perform activities of daily living. Additionally she reported Raynaud's phenomenon, debilitating fatigue, unexplained fevers and proximal muscle ache.

Physical examination was completely unremarkable except for severe swelling and tenderness in the metacarpophalangeal (MCP) and proximal interphalangeal (PIP) joints and completely reducible Jaccoud's deformities. Laboratory evaluations included slightly low Hb and albumin, slightly high total globulin count, normal platelet count, normal urinalysis and an ESR of 80 mm/h. Anti-CCP antibody was moderately positive at 48 U/ml, rheumatoid factor was positive at 137 IU/ml (cutoff 80). ANA, performed by IFA on Hep-2 cell line, was positive with a nuclear speckled pattern at 1:29,160. Nuclear RNP antibody was positive by ouchterlony. CH50 was markedly low (8/50). An MRI of her hands was performed (**25a** [with contrast], **25b** [T1]).

25a

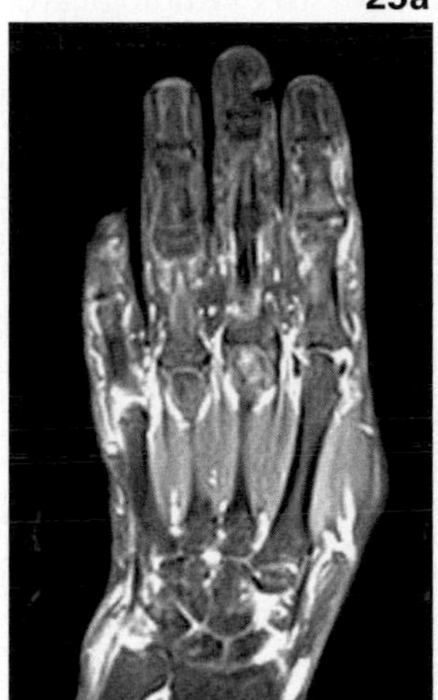

25b

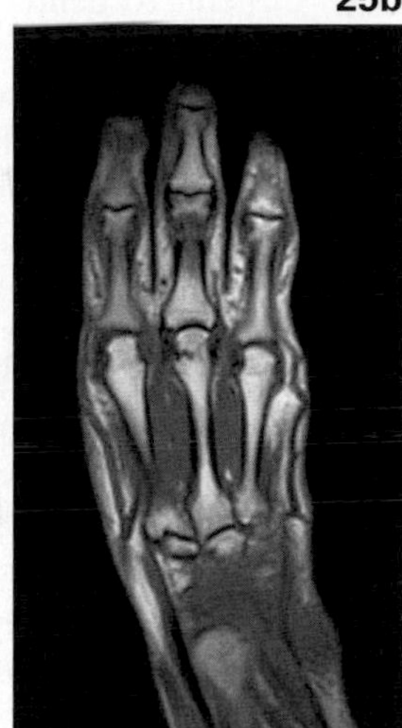

Questions

1 What do the MRIs show?
2 What is the diagnosis?
3 How should the patient be managed?

CASE 24

Answers

1 Neck pain, whether unilateral or bilateral is common in people who work under high pressure at computers. It is usually muscular and due to muscle spasm. There may be local tender trigger points in the trapezius muscle, at the upper medial scapula, over the C7 spinous process or at the occipital ridge. Neck movements are often restricted but rarely to the degree that this man demonstrates. At his age significant spondylosis on x-ray is unlikely unless he has played a lot of contact sports such as rugby. The relevance of spondylosis to neck pain is often difficult to define as it persists radiologically even if the pain resolves. Such pain is usually best called non-specific or muscular neck pain. In this patient the severity of the pain and the radiation to the interscapular region are highly suggestive of a disc prolapse, albeit without arm symptoms.

2 Analgesia, a short course of muscle relaxants for the spasm and a collar for a few days are worth trying. The patient will need to have his work station reviewed to make sure that the keyboard and screen are at the optimum position. He may need some time off work.

3 The best way to investigate the patient if the pain remains severe or if he develops arm symptoms such as pain and 'pins and needles' or weakness in a dermatomal distribution is an MRI.

Outcome

The patient developed severe left arm pain radiating to the right index finger and thumb a couple of days later. MRI scan showed a very large central and left sided disc prolapse at C5/6 (**24**). The disc was compressing the left C6 nerve root in the lateral recess and the central portion of the disc was compressing the spinal cord although there were no myelopathic changes in the cord. He was referred urgently to a neurosurgeon and underwent an urgent decompression from an anterior approach. He made an excellent recovery and is back to work and sports.

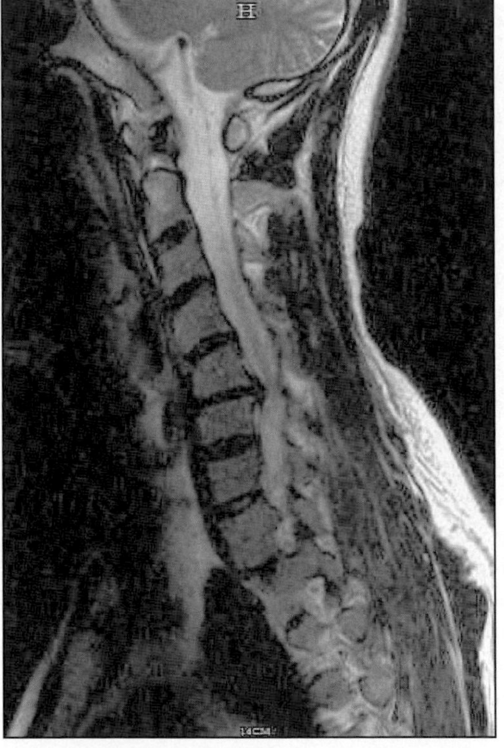

24

CASE 25

Answers

1 The first MRI image shows synovitis of the left distal radioulnar joint, and in the carpus. In addition, there is synovitis of all of the MCPs and of the index finger PIP. The second image (T1 weighted) shows an erosion affecting the third MCP of the right hand.

2 This patient meets criteria for rheumatoid arthritis (RA), but the reducible deformities and extremely high titre ANA with low CH50 and positive RNP antibody leave open the possibility of a mixed connective tissue disease. However, to date, she does not meet criteria for systemic lupus erythematosus (SLE).

3 Continue to monitor her for any signs of insidious organ flares beyond what might be expected from RA alone. Use of a TNF inhibitor might also be approached cautiously, given the possibility that this might trigger an SLE flare.

CASE 26

A 14-year-old girl with polyarticular juvenile idiopathic arthritis (JIA) came to the clinic for three-monthly review. She was on sulphasalazine (SPZ) 1 g bd and methotrexate (MTX) 20 mg/week subcutaneously. In the preceding 12 months, the SPZ had been started, and the MTX dose increased. She was very anxious about the development of numerous small lumps on her hands (**26a, 26b**).

Questions

1 What do the images show?
2 What are they caused by?
3 How should the patient be managed now?
4 What are the advantages of subcutaneous MTX in the management of JIA?

26a

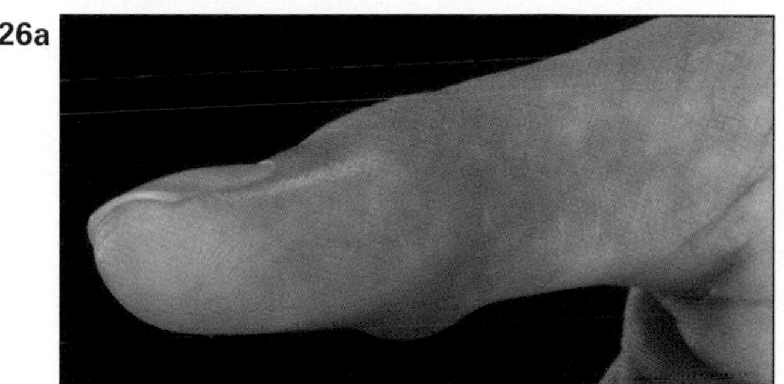

26b

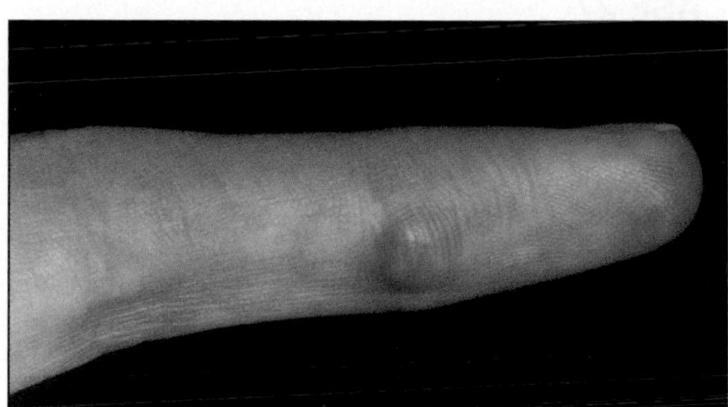

CASE 27

A 55-year-old refugee from the Balkans came to the clinic. She has permanent leave to stay and lives with her two teenage children but speaks no English. She had been in the UK for 10 years. She was badly treated by her ex-husband and by the police. She complained of a 10-year history of bilateral lower back pain which was constant and limits her activity. Her children did most of the housework and shopping although she struggled to do what she could. She spent a lot of time resting on her bed. She slept badly and appeared depressed but smiled when she reported that her children were doing well at school. On questioning she also had pain around the base of the neck, chronic bifrontal headaches and pain in the limbs and described 'too much pain all over my body'. Her weight was steady. She complained of bloating and abdominal pain which had been diagnosed as irritable bowel syndrome. There was little to find on examination. She was not especially tender anywhere but apprehensive.

Questions

1 What is the likely diagnosis?
2 What tests would help to support your diagnosis?
3 What is the best way to mange this patient?

CASE 26

ANSWERS

1 Methotrexate nodulosis.
2 Introduction of MTX therapy, or increasing the dose, in someone who is rheumatoid factor positive.
3 Reduction of the MTX dose, and introduction of an alternative DMARD/TNF inhibitor (see table of drug options in Appendix 2).
4 Adherence to treatment can be a real problem, particularly in teenagers. Subcutaneous injections allow for careful monitoring of drug administration. In addition nausea related to MTX is a particular problem among patients with JIA, and this often improves when MTX is switched from oral to subcutaneous form.

CASE 27

ANSWERS

1 Although it is necessary to exclude any inflammatory cause the most likely diagnosis from the history is of what is now usually called chronic widespread pain (previously fibromyalgia). Some tests are appropriate both to reassure you that you are not missing something more serious but also to help the patient to understand that they are being taken seriously. Although tender trigger points are necessary to diagnose fibromyalgia, they are not always present in chronic widespread pain.

The combination of depression, irritable bowel syndrome and tension headaches (and sometimes urinary urgency and premenstrual syndrome) are all suggestive of what is often called a wind-up or hypervigilance syndrome. The importance of the first description of fibromyalgia was that it established a recognized (albeit still not by everyone) syndrome in patients who had chronic unexplained pain. Previously it was all too easy to 'blame' the patient and expect them to 'pull themselves together'. There is now experimental evidence that there is overactivity of the CNS and a failure of the normal descending inhibition which allows us normally, for example, to read a book and shut out the radio.
2 A basic blood screen (blood count, thyroid function, vitamin D) and possibly some x-rays or a bone scan will help to exclude more sinister causes, although the length of history makes these unlikely. It may help to discuss the results with the help of a medical interpreter rather than depending on the children to translate what are often difficult concepts.
3 Reassurance and explanation are essential. It is important not to imply that the pain has no cause, merely that it has no serious or progressive cause and is likely to be the result of a long period of stress and distress. Sleeplessness or poor sleep quality are central to the problem and treatment with low doses of amitriptyline, not as an antidepressant but as a sedative and slow acting pain reliever, is often helpful. Side-effects such as morning dopiness and a dry mouth can be a problem but are minimized by a gradual increase in the dose. Adequate simple analgesia is also important – paracetamol in full dose or with a small amount of codeine. Stronger morphine-like derivatives are best avoided. Cognitive behavioural therapy and gentle graded exercises under supervision help if the patient has sufficient English to manage working in a group.

Outcome

The patient was treated with low doses of amitriptyline (5 mg gradually increasing to 25 mg) taken 2 hours before bed. She began to sleep better. The initial 6 months were difficult as she was convinced that she had cancer. By a careful series of consultations and because she eventually accepted that the tests, including an MRI of the spine, were all normal she began to come to terms with her pain and to manage it better. Although group cognitive behavioural therapy was not possible because of language difficulties she attended several sessions with a psychologist, including one with her children. They began to be more sympathetic and not to do everything for her and she began to mix with neighbours. Six years later she now speaks English and is managing well.

CASE 28

A 71-year-old retired shopkeeper presented to the rheumatology clinic with a 2-month history of an inflammatory polyarthritis affecting the small joints of his hands, wrists and knees. He had early morning stiffness of 2 hours, and gross synovitis on examination. His rheumatoid factor and anti-CCP antibodies were strongly positive. The diagnosis of seropositive rheumatoid arthritis was made.

On further questioning he admitted to a 12-month history of increasing breathlessness. A chest x-ray was performed (**28a**). Pulmonary function tests demonstrated a restrictive defect with a transfer factor of 41% predicted.

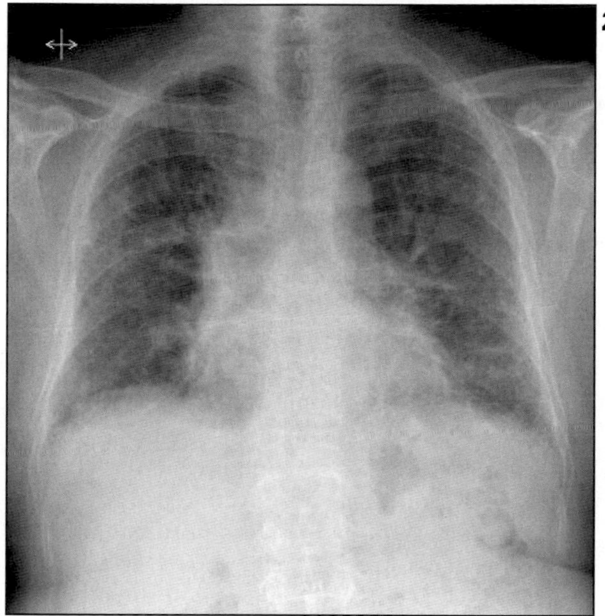

28a

Questions

1 What does the chest x-ray show?
2 What further investigations are required?
3 How should the patient's arthritis be managed?

CASE 29

A 37-year-old bartender slipped on an icy pavement and fell onto his left buttock while walking home one night. He was able to get up and make his way home, but by the following morning, he noticed pain and soreness in the mid buttock region. There was no bruising however. Over ensuing days, the pain persisted. He began to experience numbness in the posterior left thigh radiating down to the bottom of the foot. Pressure on the mid buttock exacerbated his pain. He found it difficult to sit or climb stairs.

On examination of his lumbar spine, there was no focal tenderness and he had full pain-free range of movement. Straight leg raised to 80° produced no discomfort bilaterally.

On examination of the left hip, there was no tenderness over the greater trochanter. External rotation to 40° produced some discomfort. Internal rotation to 10° produced discomfort. On the right, internal rotation was 35° and external rotation 45°. Palpation over the left sciatic notch reproduced the pain and numbness. Plain x-rays of the hip were normal.

Question

What is the most likely diagnosis?

CASE 28

ANSWERS

1 Bilateral reticular shadowing can be observed, predominantly in the mid and lower zones, consistent with interstitial lung disease.

2 High resolution CT scan of the chest is required. This was done and demonstrated a combination of usual interstitial pneumonitis and non-specific interstitial pneumonitis. The CT scan (**28b**) shows both honeycombing and some ground-glass shadowing. There remains coarse, widespread fibrosis with architectural distortion and honeycombing throughout all lobes. It has a lower lobe predominance. If anything, there has been a slight improvement as some inflammatory changes in the middle lobe have improved.

3 The presence of pulmonary fibrosis precludes the use of methotrexate, leflunomide or probably the anti-TNF agents. Steroids can be used, but are clearly not a long-term solution. Sulphasalazine and hydroxychloroquine could be used, but given the aggressive nature of his arthritis, he was given rituximab.

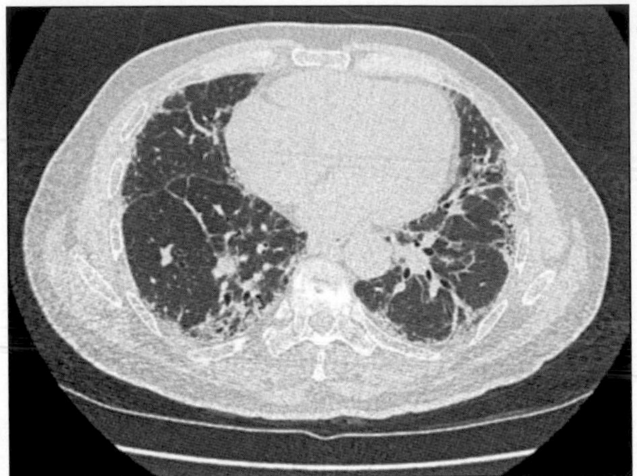

28b

CASE 29

ANSWER

Left piriformis syndrome is indicated. The syndrome is caused by irritation of the sciatic nerve as it passes below or through the piriformis muscle, which is an abductor and external rotator of the thigh. Common findings include tenderness over the sciatic notch and loss of internal rotation on the affected side. This syndrome is often mistakenly diagnosed as sciatica, which is a radiculopathy arising from compression of the sciatic nerve roots at the level of the lumbar spine.

Treatment involves rest in the acute phase, anti-inflammatories and stretching exercises as symptoms improve. The syndrome often recurs after the initial event.

CASE 30

A 42-year-old man with HIV was known to the rheumatology department because of two previous episodes of reactive arthritis following a gonococcal urethritis. This had responded well to treatment. He re-presented 2 years later with pain in his left hip and left knee. This time, there were no other features of Reiter's syndrome. His CD4 count was 400 μl, and his viral load was low.

On examination, there was no synovitis. Movement of the knees were normal, but movement of the left hip was markedly reduced in all directions, and produced considerable pain. Bloods revealed a normal CRP and ESR.

An x-ray of his pelvis was taken (**30a**).

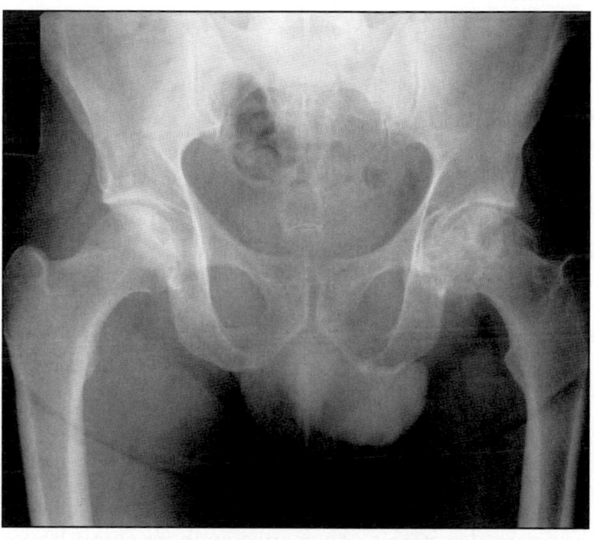

30a

Questions

1 What does the x-ray show?
2 What are the likely causes?
3 What is the knee pain due to?
4 What is the management?

CASE 31

A 56-year-old Caucasian woman was referred with a history of lower back pain and persistently raised ALP. Preliminary blood tests had shown a normal full blood count, ALP of 170 IU/l and a normal GGT.

Four years earlier she noticed a dull persistent ache and early morning stiffness in the thighs. The pain lasted about 3 weeks then resolved spontaneously. Six months later, she noticed onset of lower back pain, which was non-radiating, worse in the mornings and aggravated by turning in bed or standing for long periods. She had lost 5 kg over 6 months and her appetite was poor. There was no history of fever or night sweats. She had no symptoms referable to the bowels, urinary tract, or cardiorespiratory system.

Seven weeks ago, she noticed recurrence of thigh aches and aches in the shoulders especially on trying to comb her hair. There was no loss of muscle strength and no joint swelling. On examination, she was tender over T12–L3. Flexion of the spine to 60° caused discomfort. The remainder of the examination was normal.

Questions

1 What are the differential diagnoses?
2 What investigations might be indicated in this patient?

CASE 30

ANSWERS

1 The film shows avascular necrosis (AVN) or osteonecrosis.
2 HIV and some antiretrovirals are risk factors for AVN. In addition, he had had two 3–6 month courses of corticosteroids for management of reactive arthritis.
3 His knee pain was referred from his hip, and completely resolved after left total hip replacement.
4 He was immediately non-weight bearing and seen by the orthopaedic surgeons for an urgent total hip replacement. He was also screened for AVN elsewhere.

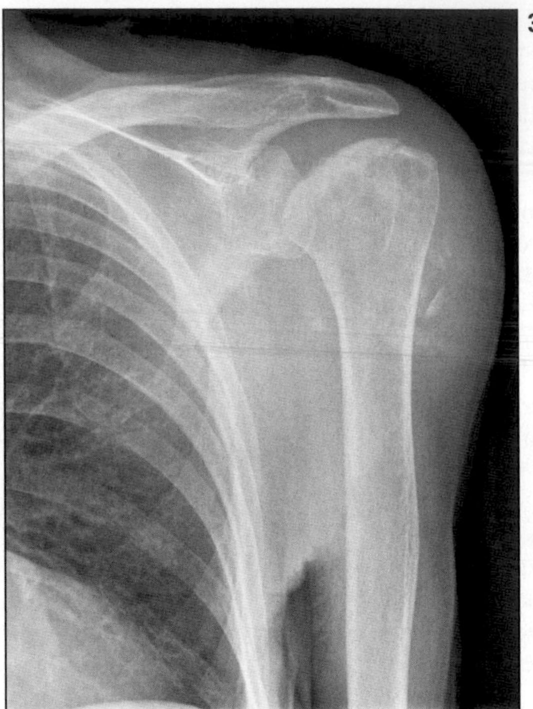

30b

Discussion

AVN most commonly affects the femoral head, but can also affect other sites such as small bones of hands and feet, tibia and humeral head. **Figure 30b** shows AVN of the left humeral head in an elderly lady on long-term steroid use for chronic obstructive pulmonary disease.

Table 30 shows other rheumatological manifestations/complications of HIV.

Table 30 Other rheumatological manifestations/complications of HIV

HIV-associated arthritis or arthralgia	Increased risk of septic arthritis
Reactive arthritis	Vasculitis
Psoriatic arthritis	Lupus-like syndrome
Viral myositis	Sjögren's-like syndrome

CASE 31

ANSWERS

1 Causes of a raised ALP and proximal muscle aches should be considered including: osteomalacia, malignancies, Paget's disease, primary hyperparathyroidism, polymyalgia rheumatica and infection involving bone. Two or more coexisting pathologies may explain her symptoms, e.g. osteoarthritis in combination with any of the above, thyroid dysfunction (proximal muscle aches) and bony fractures.

2 The following may help to clarify the diagnosis: ESR, CRP, vitamin D, repeat liver function tests, immunoglobulins, serum protein electrophoresis, urine Bence Jones proteins, muscle enzymes including CK, parathyroid hormone, calcium, phosphate, magnesium, thyroid function tests, urinary hydroxyproline, x-rays of thoracolumbar spine, bone scan and chest x-ray.

CASE 32

A 49-year-old woman of mixed African and Caucasian descent presented to clinic with a several month history of patchy alopecia and rash on her scalp, recently biopsied and confirmed to be discoid lupus. A full review of systems was negative for any other findings other than chronic migraine headaches.

Laboratory investigations were completely normal except for a positive ANA at 1:160 and low CH50 and low C4.

She was well for the next 18 months when she suddenly developed some new discoid lesions with tenderness and a pressure sensation of the scalp, accompanied by sores of the buccal mucosa that lasted several weeks. At this visit, a full history revealed new onset of bilateral, symmetrical arthralgia, proximal myalgia, recent onset of Raynaud's phenomenon, unexplained fevers and fatigue. These symptoms responded to a short course of steroids.

For the next 9 months she was well except for occasional mild flares of her scalp lesions which were controlled with hydroxychloroquine.

She then developed a syndrome of moderately severe fatigue, fevers, loss of appetite, low grade nausea, muscle aches and polyarticular inflammatory arthritis with morning stiffness for 1 hour and swelling in fingers, elbows, knees, ankles and toes. This responded promptly to prednisone, 40 mg PO od. For the first time, laboratory workup demonstrated a positive anti-cardiolipin antibody along with a positive ANA and persistently low complement studies.

Questions

1 Is this a typical presentation of systemic lupus erythematosus (SLE)?
2 Was it expected to occur in this case?

CASE 33

A 50-year-old woman presented with a 16-month history of left sided pelvic pain. The pains were present at rest, exacerbated by movement, and seemed to be worse at night, interfering with her sleep. There was no history of fever, night sweats or weight loss. Her past medical history included a cholecystectomy 5 years ago. Blood tests revealed normal FBC, ESR, urea, creatinine and electrolytes, serum calcium, phosphate and albumin. The ALT, AST and GGT were normal. The ALP was three times the upper limit of normal. An x-ray of her pelvis is shown (**33a**).

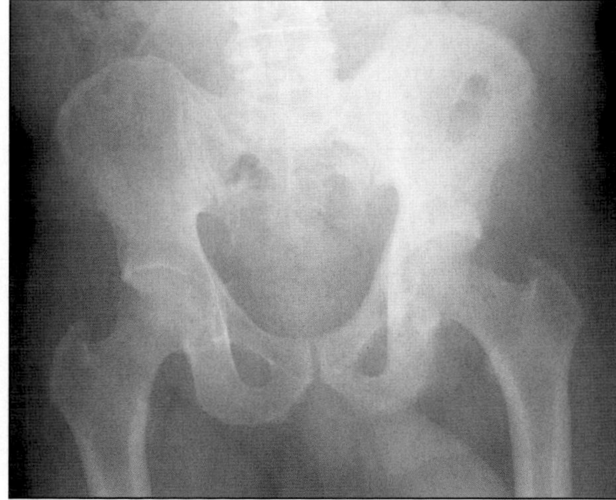

33a

Questions

1 What is the most likely diagnosis?
2 What other investigations might be helpful in the patient's further management?
3 What is the aetiology of this condition?
4 How should the patient be treated?
5 What musculoskeletal neoplastic conditions might be associated with this condition?

CASE 32

ANSWERS

1 About 10% of patients with primary discoid lupus erythematosus (LE) will progress to develop systemic lupus.

2 A presentation with discoid LE, restricted to the scalp, at the age of 49 years would not suggest a high likelihood of such progression. This patient did evolve over several years to meet criteria for SLE, but to date has exhibited a milder form, restricted to cutaneous and musculoskeletal manifestations, although she has had discrete episodes of generalized systemic illness. A higher index of suspicion might have been elicited earlier if her skin lesions had progressed both above and below the neck.

CASE 33

ANSWERS

1 The x-ray identifies Paget's disease of the bone. The radiographic features of Paget's disease are considered pathognomonic. Paget's disease is a disorder of bone remodelling. The primary abnormality is in osteoclast-mediated bone resorption. Increased bone resorption appears as a decrease in density of the bone and osteolytic areas. Older lesions may have a mixed sclerotic and lytic appearance.

2 A bone scan and x-rays of painful bones are the next step to determine the extent of the disease. The isotope bone scan of this patient is shown here (**33b**). Biochemical indices of bone resorption including deoxypyridinoline and peptides of the cross-linking domains of collagen type 1 such as the urine N-telopeptide or the serum C-telopeptide may confirm accelerated bone resorption, the extent and severity of the disease and are also useful for monitoring response to treatment.

3 Genetic factors are thought to play a role. Studies report a seven to tenfold increased risk of the disease in first-degree relatives. A possible infectious aetiology has been supported by the finding of viral particles in the nuclei and cytoplasm of osteoclasts in Paget's disease. Paramyxoviruses, the measles virus and the dog distemper virus have been implicated.

4 Bone pain is an indication for active treatment. Oral bisphosphonates such as risedronate are usually effective. Treatment doses and protocols vary. Intravenous bisphosphonates such as pamidronate or zoledronic acid are useful in patients who are not able to tolerate oral preparations or who fail to respond to oral bisphosphonates. A response is marked by resolution of pain, and a fall in bone resorption markers followed by ALP. Treatment may be repeated if the patient relapses. Salmon calcitonin given subcutaneously is beneficial in treating Pagetic bone pain, hearing loss and neurological complications. Gallium nitrate given cyclically is effective in polyostotic Paget's, but renal failure is a side-effect.

5 Sarcomas including osteosarcomas, fibrosarcomas and chondrosarcomas may occur but are generally rare (incidence of less than 1%). Giant cell tumours (mostly benign) may also occur.

33b

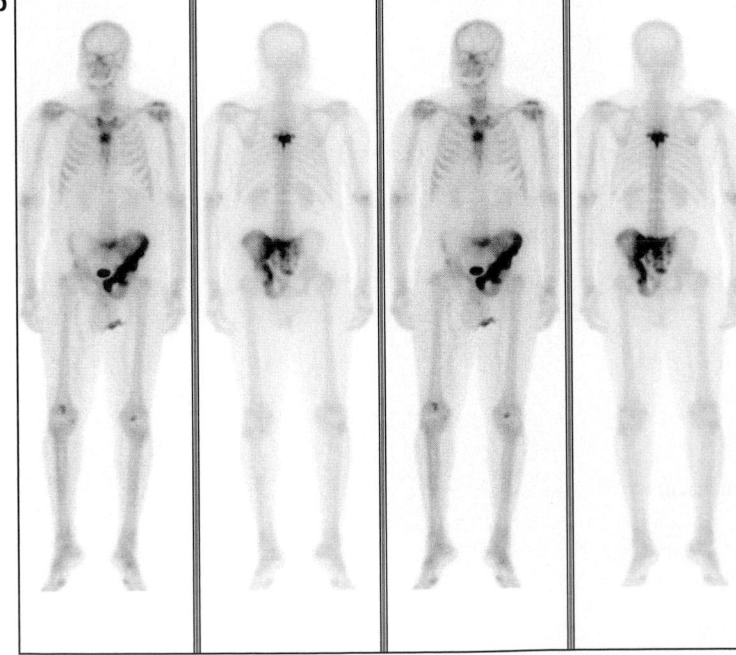

CASE 34

A 69-year-old man presented to the emergency department with a 2-day history of a rash affecting his hands and feet (**34a, 34b**). He had been diagnosed with seropositive rheumatoid arthritis (RA) 5 years earlier, and his disease had been difficult to manage. The rash was associated with a flare of his arthritis. Investigations are shown in *Table 34*.

Treatment was initiated, but on day 3 of his admission the patient developed chest pain. He had no history of ischaemic heart disease. An ECG was performed (**34c**).

Questions

1 What is the diagnosis?
2 How should this be managed?

34a

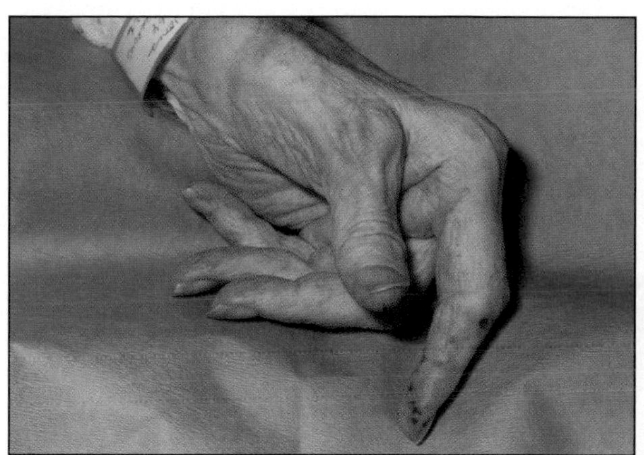

34b

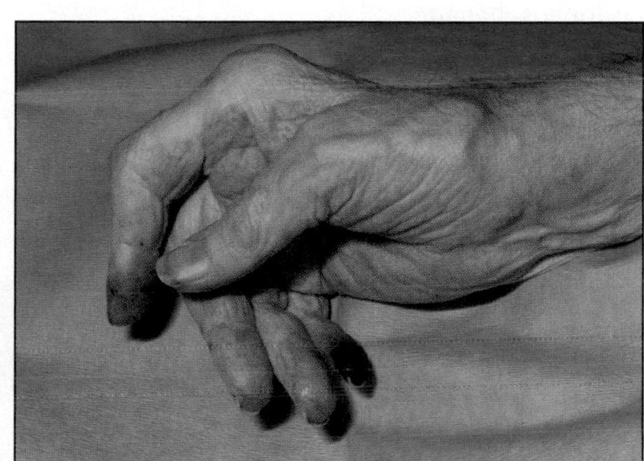

Table 34 Results of investigation

Hb	10.2 g/dl	Urea	7.8 mmol/l
WBC	8.4 x 10^9/l	Creat	110 μmol/l
Plt	560 x 10^9/l	ANCA	Negative
Albumin	32 g/l	ANA	Negative
ALT	38 IU/l	Cryoglobulins	Negative
Bilirubin	16 μmol/l	Urinalysis	Normal
ALP	100 IU/l		

34c

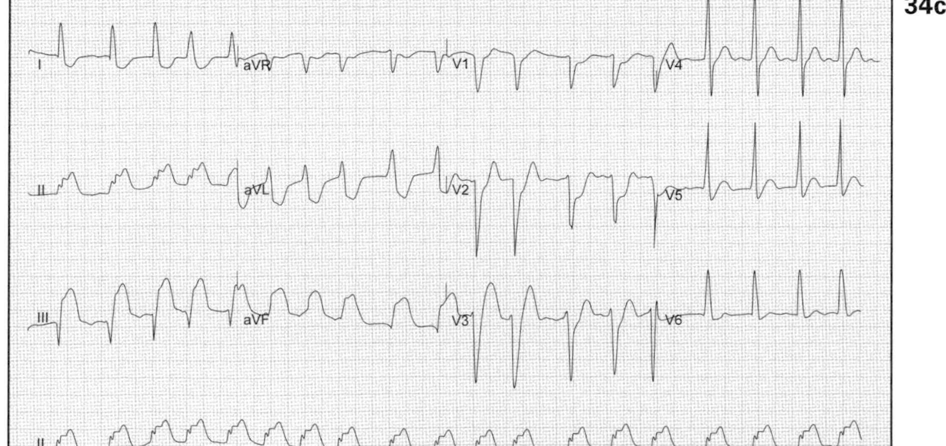

(Courtesy of Azeem *et al.* [2005] *Rapid Review of ECG Interpretation*, CRC Press.)

CASE 34

Answers

1 The patient has rheumatoid vasculitis, complicated by coronary angiitis. This is a rare complication of RA which affects men and women equally. Often it causes only a cutaneous vasculitis, but there is a poor prognosis associated with renal or cardiac involvement.

2 No good trials exist, but it is generally managed with corticosteroids and if necessary cyclophosphamide.

Outcome

The patient was treated aggressively with IV methylprednisolone and cyclophosphamide, but despite this and a transfer to ITU, he died 5 days later. He had ignored the skin lesions for many weeks as he thought they were from self-testing his glucose levels.

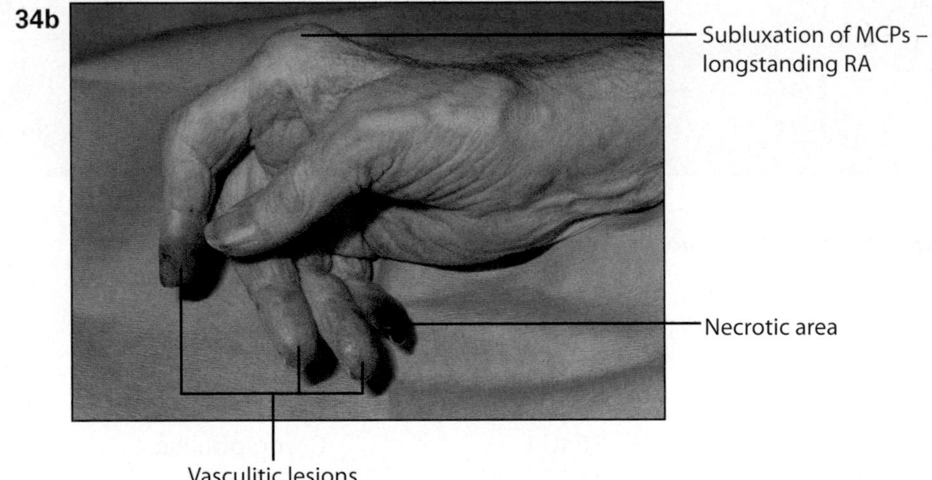

CASE 35

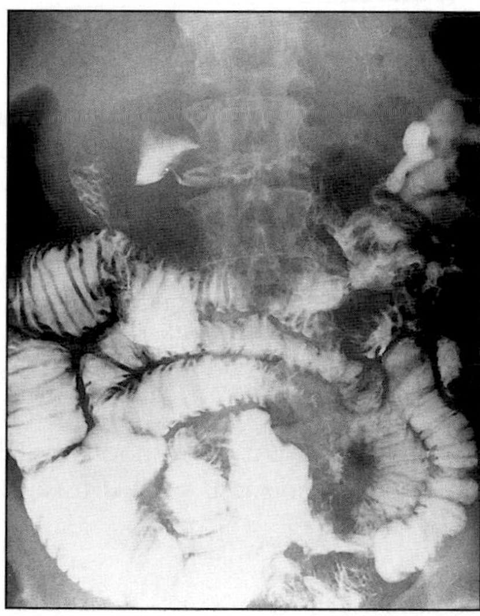
35

A woman aged 45 years presented to the emergency department complaining of severe pain in her fingers. On examination they were blue but just as noticeably her skin was tightly drawn over the fingers and this skin tightness extended to the mid forearm. Further history taking revealed a history of Raynaud's phenomenon for 2 years. She had tried to cope by increasing her dietary intake of fish oils (she had a great reluctance to take any kind of medication) and this has given her some relief.

During systemic questioning she mentioned that her appetite had been poor, that she had lost some weight, around 5 kg, and that she was increasingly constipated.

On examination, apart from the skin thickening there was evidence of early telangiectasia over her face, and her abdomen was little distended.

Investigations showed Hb of 10.9 g/dl with iron deficient indices. Urea and electrolytes and liver function tests were normal. An ultrasound examination confirmed the presence of some distended bowel loops and a barium enema was undertaken (35).

Questions

1 What distinguishes the thickening of the skin seen in patients with scleroderma and those with eosinophilic fasciitis?
2 Assuming that her anti-nuclear antibody test was positive what fine specificity might be anticipated?
3 What abnormality does the barium enema show?
4 Although an extreme measure, what therapeutic endeavour might well be needed?
5 Is the large bowel the only part of the gastro-intestinal tract likely to be involved in scleroderma?

CASE 36

A 29-year-old Turkish man presented to his primary care physician complaining of recurrent painful genital ulcers, joint aches and fatigue for over 6 months. In the past 3 months he had noticed a few painful oral ulcers but assumed that these ulcers were caused by a new brand of toothpaste which he had been using. He denied any photosensitivity, eye problems, Raynaud's symptoms, sicca symptoms, joint swelling, penile discharge or bowel symptoms. He had noticed two small, tender erythematous firm lumps over his left shin a few weeks ago but these had resolved with no intervention.

His primary care physician requested blood tests including ANA, dsDNA antibodies, RF, HLA-B27, coeliac screen, B12, folate and iron studies, all of which returned negative or normal. A full sexually transmitted infection screen including tests for HIV and herpes simplex 1 returned negative. Throat swab revealed normal flora. His ESR was elevated at 38 mm/h with a CRP of 13 mg/l.

When he returned to see his primary care physician 2 days later for review she noticed that a pustule had formed at the site of the pinprick (phlebotomy site). She then referred him on to a rheumatologist for review.

Three years later he developed insidious left lower limb pain and swelling. Doppler ultrasound confirmed a proximal deep vein thrombosis (DVT). Blood tests revealed normal protein C, protein S and antithrombin 111 levels. Anticardiolipin, serum B2GP1 and lupus anticoagulant tests were also negative. He was treated with heparin followed by warfarin. Within 3 months there was clinical and sonographic resolution of the DVT.

Questions

1 What condition is likely in this patient and how might he be treated?
2 How common are venous thrombotic events in patients with this condition?

CASE 35

Answers

1 Patients with eosinophilic fasciitis usually have involvement of the forearm without involvement of the skin over the hands, which is a hallmark of scleroderma. In addition, Raynaud's phenomenon while invariably found in patients with scleroderma is rare in eosinophilic fasciitis.

2 Given the relative restricted nature of the skin involvement this patient is more likely to be anti-centromere positive and anti-topoisomerase-1 negative. The latter antibody, also known as anti-SCL70, is associated with diffuse skin disease and accompanying renal and lung disease. However, gut involvement is more common in diffuse disease.

3 The imaging shows significantly distended loops of large bowel almost certainly affected by her scleroderma.

4 Excision of the affected portion of the bowel might be necessary.

5 Scleroderma may affect the gastrointestinal tract from mouth to anus with the lower end of the oesophagus being the most commonly affected part, with reflux oesophagitis and stricture.

CASE 36

Answers

1 Behçet's disease is the likely diagnosis. He presents with recurrent painful oral and genital ulcers and a positive pathergy test (cutaneous hypersensitivity to trauma) which are three of the classification criteria put forward by the International Study Group for Behçet's disease which aid in diagnosis of this condition. Oral ulceration is a mandatory clinical feature. His description of firm, tender erythematous lumps on the legs is suggestive of erythema nodosum which is also associated with this condition. Initial treatment might involve the use of oral colchicine, oral corticosteroids and steroid based mouth washes.

2 Venous thromboses are the most frequent vascular manifestation of Behçet's disease and may be seen in up to 33% of cases. They occur most often in males and in patients who have a positive pathergy test. In the majority of instances, DVT events occur within 3 years after the diagnosis of Behçet's. Thrombosis appears to be due to vasculitis rather than to a clotting disorder.

Venous thromboses most commonly affect the lower limbs but may also involve the venae cavae. Hepatic venous thrombosis is a rare complication occurring in less than 1% of cases, but may be fatal.

CASE 37

A 42-year-old Caucasian-Hispanic woman with systemic lupus erythematosus (SLE) noticed progressively yellow eyes, weakness and swelling in her body over a several week period.

The patient had been in good health until the age of 40 years when she developed Coombs positive haemolytic anaemia while pregnant. This responded to transfusions and prednisone, but subsequently redeveloped after her child was born, when a steroid taper was attempted. Eventually she received four doses of rituximab and was well for more than 1 year off steroids without incident.

She then presented with a mild/moderate photosensitive, hyperpigmented rash, recurrent bouts of mild oral ulcers, leucopenia/lymphopenia, positive ANA, anti-dsDNA and anti-cardiolipin antibodies. She had other suggestive features of lupus as well, including low C4, marked livedo reticularis, Raynaud's phenomenon, sicca symptoms and polyarticular arthralgias, although there was no objective synovitis. Hydroxychloroquine 200 mg bd was prescribed with a good response of all symptoms.

At the current visit she returned to the clinic describing general malaise, swollen extremities and yellow discolouration in her eyes. On review of systems she had worsening fatigue, and swelling in legs, trunk and around her eyes, which was apparently worse in the morning. C3 values had dropped to below normal and her anti-dsDNA titre had risen.

She had mild livedo reticularis and active Raynaud's phenomenon which were the same as usual. There were no other active findings on review of systems or physical examination. Labs were remarkable for a WBC count of 3.5×10^9/l and absolute lymphocyte count of 0.38×10^9/l. Creatinine clearance was 69 ml/min, urinalysis was unremarkable and hour urine protein was 81 mg/24 h. Coombs test was positive, and Hb had dropped from 10.7 to 8.9 g/dl. Soon after this value was reported, she was admitted to the hospital with Hb that had dropped to 6.2 g/dl.

Question

What causes anaemia in lupus and how is it the best treated?

CASE 38

An 84-year-old woman with long-standing rheumatoid arthritis complained of worsening neck pain. There was no radiation to arms or legs, and neurology examination was unremarkable. Her flexion (**38a**) and extension (**38b**) films are shown.

Questions

Describe the findings.

38a

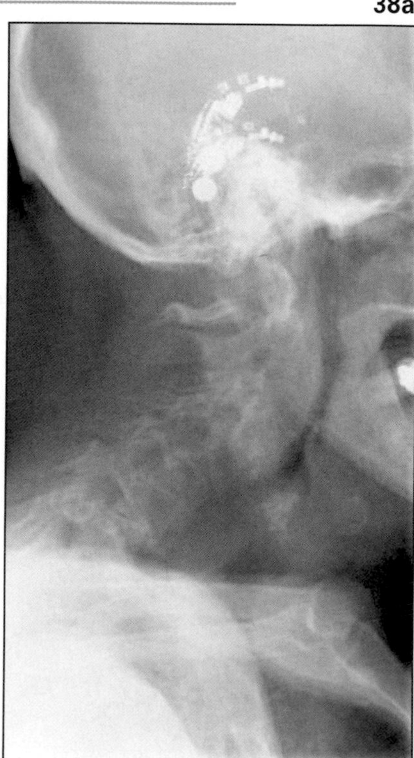

38b

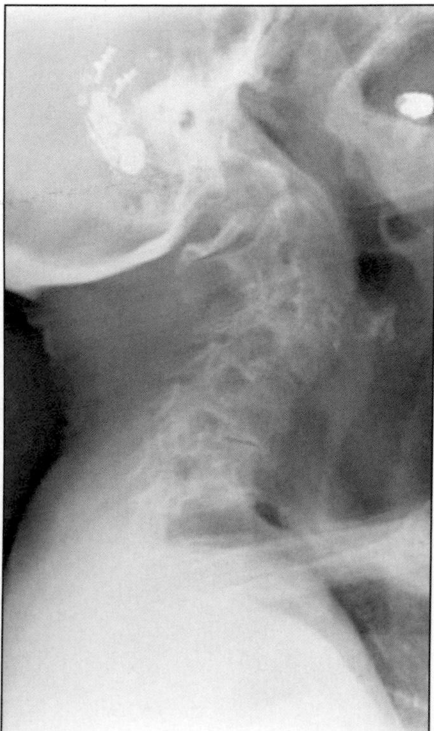

CASE 37

Answer

The most common cause of anaemia in lupus patients is anaemia of chronic disease, characterized by decreased bone marrow production of red cells, probably in response to inflammatory signals. This anaemia can be chronic, but may sometimes respond to more aggressive disease control. Anaemia can also be caused by iron deficiency, particularly in this largely female population, and/or renal disease. This patient has haemolytic anaemia which may affect roughly 5% of lupus patients. Haemolytic anaemia usually responds rapidly to steroids, but alternative treatments may be needed to spare steroid use in refractory cases.

CASE 38

Answer

There is generalized reduction in bone density. There is subluxation of about 30% of C4/5 and minimal subluxation at C5/6. Fusion of the C6/7 disc and further subluxation of about 30% C7/D1 can be seen. The facet joints are all narrowed and possibly fused. There is no atlantoaxial subluxation. (Hearing aids are noted.)

CASE 39

This patient suffered from prominent Raynaud's symptoms.

QUESTIONS

1 What striking features are shown in the x-ray of the patient's hands (39)?
2 What is the likely diagnosis?

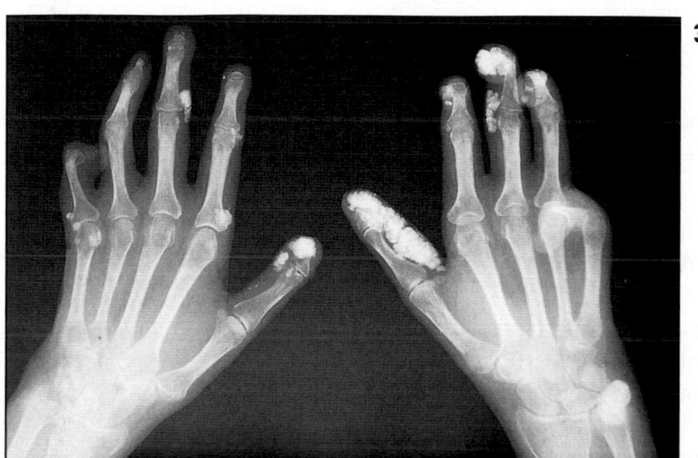

39

CASE 40

A 64-year-old woman was referred by the oncology department. She had undergone mastectomy and radiotherapy for carcinoma of the breast 5 years earlier, and had no evidence of disease recurrence. She gave a 6-month history of joint pains. She described pain in a variety of joints, always one at a time. The most common joints were both wrists, the interphalangeal (IP) joints of the thumbs and the ankles. The pain would come on fairly suddenly, ascend to a peak of fairly severe pain, and settle over the next 5 days. The pain was associated with redness and some swelling of the affected joint. She took ibuprofen 200 mg intermittently, which helped a bit.

At the time of the review, all her joints looked normal. Blood tests showed CRP 6 mg/l, ESR 12 mm/h, negative rheumatoid factor (RF) and urate 320 μmol/l.

QUESTIONS

1 What is the differential diagnosis?
2 How should the patient be managed?

CASE 39

Answers
1 Calcinosis and resorption of phalanges
2 Scleroderma.

CASE 40

Answers
1 The differential diagnoses include gout, pseudogout and palindromic rheumatism. Against gout is the normal urate, thought this does not exclude the condition. Palindromic rheumatism is often associated with elevated inflammatory markers at the time of an attack, but between acute episodes, CRP and ESR are likely to be normal. The normal RF is also not against the diagnosis of palindromic rheumatism. Some patients, particularly those with a positive RF, go on to develop rheumatoid arthritis.
2 The patient should be seen during an acute attack so that the joint can be aspirated to look for crystals. Strong NSAIDs will reduce the pain in palindromic rheumatism, and the length of the attack in gout. Colchicine can also be used in gout or pseudogout, and corticosteroids in all three conditions. DMARDs are used in palindromic rheumatism, but there is no good evidence to support this practice.

Outcome
The patient was seen during a flare affecting the left wrist (**40**), and calcium pyrophosphate crystals were aspirated from the joint, confirming the diagnosis of pseudogout.

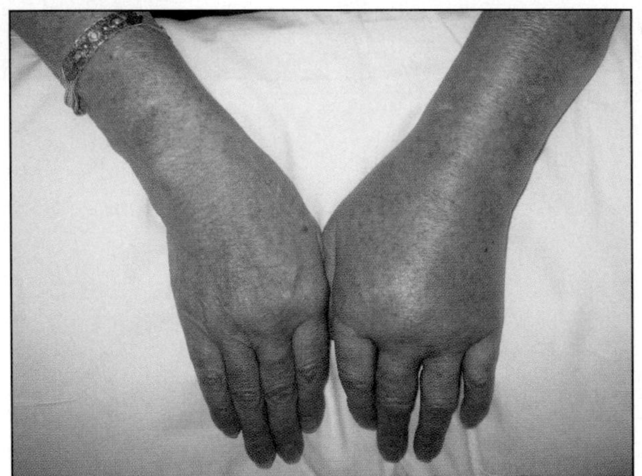
40

CASE 41

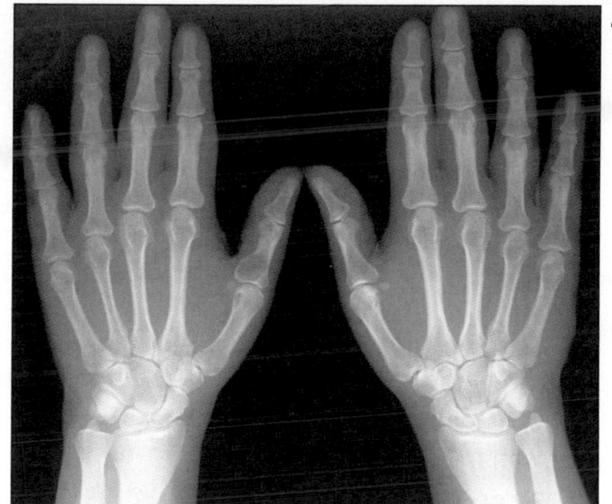
41

A 35-year-old woman came to the rheumatology clinic with a 10-month history of pain at the base of the left thumb. She described an intermittent mild, but troubling ache. On examination, she was non-tender. There was slight loss of thenar muscle bulk. The x-ray of her hands is shown (**41**).

Questions

1 What does the x-ray show and what is the diagnosis?
2 How should this be managed?

CASE 42

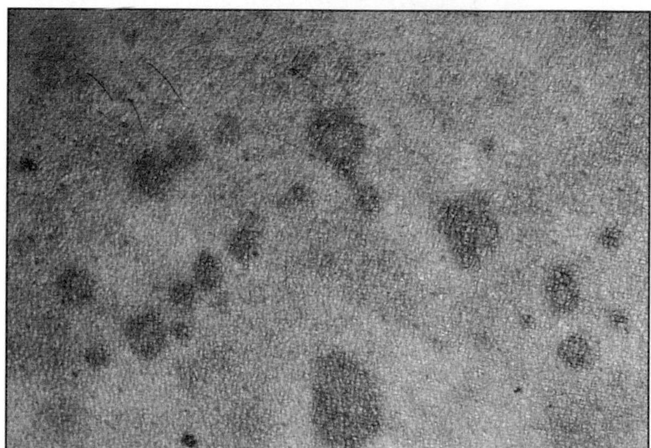
42

(Courtesy of St John's Institute of Dermatology [King's College], Guy's Hospital, London; from: Rycroft *et al.* [2010] *Dermatology, a Colour Handbook*, CRC Press.)

A 36-year-old woman presented with a history of right knee and left ankle pain. She had been previously well with no rheumatic complaints. Three months previously she had been on a 7-day camping trip to Minnesota with her church group. While there, she recalled noticing a mildly pruritic, erythematous papule on her left arm. She thought this was a mosquito bite. The papule had gradually become flat, and surrounded by marked erythema with central clearing. At the time, she felt vaguely unwell with a mild headache and some nausea. The rash slowly faded over 10 days (**42**).

Three weeks after returning to the UK, she felt lethargic with headaches, difficulty concentrating, arthralgia and mild neck stiffness but no photophobia. She was prescribed ibuprofen and paracetamol and recommended bed rest for 5 days.

Six weeks later her right knee became swollen and warm. She took ibuprofen for this but as the swelling subsided, the left ankle became quite painful. There was no urethritis, conjunctivitis or back pain. She denied any cardiorespiratory symptoms.

On examination, she was afebrile. There was some soft tissue swelling around the right knee and mild tenderness with restriction of flexion to 40°. The ankle was not swollen, but was painful on flexion and extension.

Blood tests showed WBC 11.9 × 10^9/l and ESR 39 mm/h. Rheumatoid factor, anti-CCP antibodies, HLA-B27 and ANA were negative. Blood cultures showed no growth after 24 hours, VDRL was negative. An aspirate of 1 ml of fluid from the knee joint revealed a WBC of 36.0 × 10^9/l, no crystals, no organisms on Gram stain and no acid fast bacilli. A chest x-ray was normal, but routine ECG showed first-degree heart block. There were no previous ECGs for comparison. An echocardiogram was normal.

Questions

1 What could be the cause of the patient's joint problems?
2 What serological tests could help to confirm this?
3 How could this disease have been prevented?

CASE 41

ANSWERS

1 The typical findings of an enchondroma – a well demarcated, expansile, lytic lesion. There is also a possible break in cortex representing a pathological fracture. This is a benign cartilaginous tumour of the bone, but there is a small incidence of malignant transformation.

2 The patient was referred for more imaging, MRI and CT, and then a surgical review. She opted to have removal even though there was no evidence of malignant change.

CASE 42

ANSWERS

1 The symptoms indicate Lyme disease. The patient has travelled to an endemic region and now presents with arthritis, a cardiac conduction abnormality on ECG and a history of a rash which could be erythema chronicum migrans.

2 Tests should be performed for IgM and IgG antibodies to *Borrelia* spp. which may be implicated in Lyme disease including *B. burgdorferi*, *B. afzelii* and *B. garinii* by ELISA with confirmation by western blot analysis. Polymerase chain reaction (PCR) may be done on blood, synovial or spinal fluid in the early stages of Lyme disease.

3 Vaccines have been developed in the USA, and although they showed varying degrees of efficacy, none are currently marketed, mainly because of low demand and negative media reports of side-effects. Antibiotic prophylaxis with doxycycline (200 mg stat) on appearance of the typical rash could have prevented progression of the disease. General preventive measures include the use of appropriate clothing, permethrin (a pesticide that can be applied to clothing), insect repellents, close inspection of the skin and showering after outdoor activities.

Outcome

Western blot confirmed a high titre of IgG antibodies to *B. burgdorferi*. She was treated with ceftriaxone 2 g/day for 14 days. Three months later she complained of persisting arthralgia and intermittent flares of mild ankle pain and swelling. She was subsequently treated with hydroxychloroquine 400 mg/day with ibuprofen as required.

CASE 43

A 70-year-old sprightly woman presented with a 2-day history of acute pain and swelling of the left knee. There was no ill health in the preceding few weeks and she was generally very well. She had been on a low dose of bendrofluazide for years because of puffy ankles. She had one previous episode of acute pain and swelling of a wrist which required NSAIDs and lasted about 3 weeks. There was a family history of 'knobbly fingers' and she had asymptomatic nodal osteoarthritis affecting the distal interphalangeal joints of several fingers. She had noticed that her thumbs had become swollen and stiff but were not painful.

On examination the knee was swollen, warm and tender. There was restricted flexion but no crepitus or instability. There were no other findings apart from the hand nodal osteoarthritis. She was not febrile. Her blood tests are shown in *Table 43*. Liver and renal function were normal for the patient's age. The x-ray of her knees is shown (**43a**).

Table 43 Blood test results

Hb	11.5 g/dl
WBC	11.0 x 10^9/l
Neutrophils	9.0 x 10^9/l
ESR	75 mm/h
CRP	125 mg/l

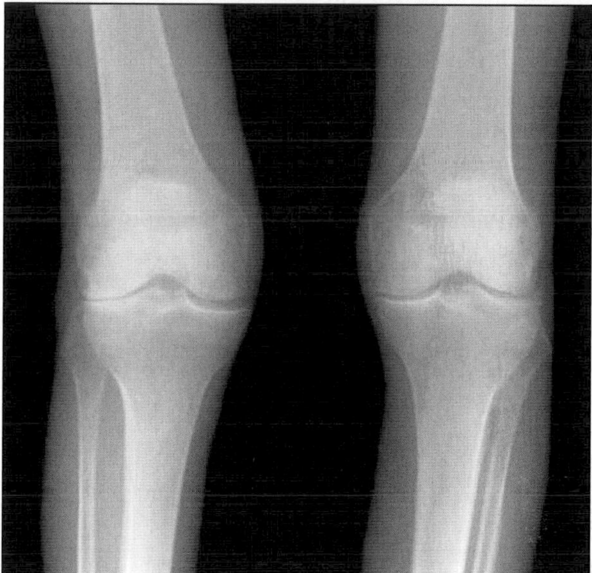

43a

Questions

1 What does the x-ray show?
2 What is the most likely diagnosis?
3 What further blood tests would you request on the stored serum sample and what is the best next investigation to perform?
4 What treatment would you recommend?

CASE 44

This patient had severe erosive rheumatoid arthritis and complains of eye pain, photophobia and tearing (**44**).

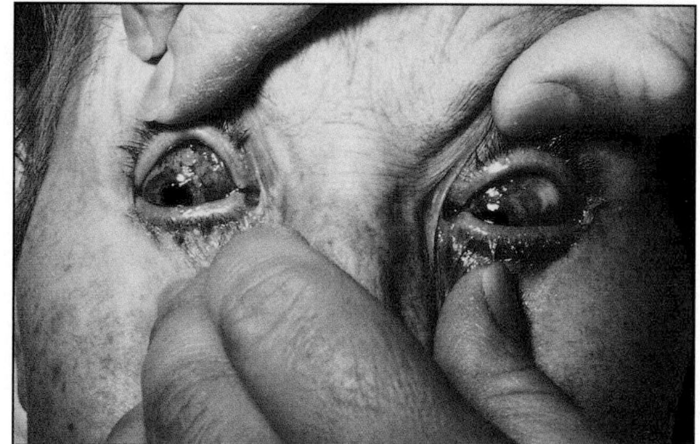

44

Question

What complication has occurred?

CASE 43

Answers

1 There is chondrocalcinosis affecting the menisci and seen as a triangular partial opacification at the medial and lateral aspects of both joints. There is a fine line of calcification just separated from the bone surface (seen in detail in **43b**). This is chondrocalcinosis in the hyaline cartilage. There are also changes of osteoarthritis.

2 The radiological appearances and the history of an acute monoarthritis first of the wrist and then of the knee in a patient over the age of 65 years suggest acute pseudogout. Gout is less likely despite the long history of bendrofluazide intake because of the joints affected. Chronic thiazide intake and/or chronic renal failure can lead to tophaceous gout and acute gout, which may be polyarticular. An acute effusion due to osteoarthritis is not likely because the knee is warm and there is no prior history of knee pain. The raised neutrophil count is not uncommon in crystal-induced arthritis.

3 The urate should be checked and may be raised. The diagnosis will be made on an aspirate from the affected knee. The fluid may be very cloudy, almost purulent, so it may be best to ask for an urgent Gram stain and polarized light microscopy before considering any steroid injection. Infection is not likely as the patient is not febrile or immunosuppressed.

4 NSAIDs and/or colchicine can be used but care needs to be taken in the elderly so assess the risk factors for peptic ulceration and adjust the dose if renal function is impaired. Sometimes it is best to use low doses (ibuprofen 400 mg tds after food or diclofenac soluble 50 mg bd after food) and colchicine 500 µg bd. Colchicine causes abdominal pain and diarrhoea if used at too high a dose. Recommend 500 µg tds for 1 day and then twice a day until the swelling and inflammation are fully controlled. Oral steroids can be used or the knee can be injected with steroid.

Outcome

The fluid was very cloudy. The patient was started on colchicine 1000 µg immediately then 500 µg tds for 3 days, then bd. The fluid contained large numbers of polymorphs, and on polarized light microscopy through a red filter there were small numbers of rhomboid shapes weakly positively birefringent crystals, some of them intracellular and diagnostic of acute pseudogout. (Urate crystals are needle shaped and strongly negatively birefringent.) Her urate was at the upper limit of normal, reflecting her chronic thiazide intake which was stopped. Culture was sterile. She made a good recovery and was advised always to carry a small supply of colchicine in case she had a recurrence.

43b

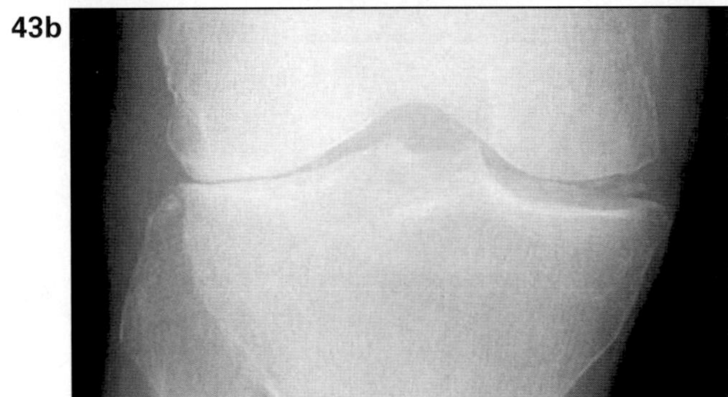

CASE 44

Answer

Nodular scleritis.

CASE 45

A 23-year-old male of Indian origin was referred to the rheumatology department with some swan neck deformities developing in his hands and a diagnosis made by his family doctor of rheumatoid arthritis (RA). On questioning in the clinic, however, other aspects of his story became evident. The hand deformities were associated with a little pain but very little, if any, swelling. The deformities had been increasing slowly over a 2- to 3-year period. In addition he had been troubled by increasing fatigue for the past 3 months and had also developed some shortness of breath with pain at the end of inspiration.

There was nothing of note in his previous medical history but in his family history he mentioned a cousin with multiple sclerosis.

On examination his pulse was 60 bpm, BP 120/87 mmHg and his heart sounds were normal. Examination of his chest revealed a left sided pleural rub. In contrast, examination of the abdomen and CNS was unremarkable. Examination of his hands revealed the deformities seen in **Figure 45**. It was notable that the deformities were correctable and that moving the joints was not painful.

Investigations included Hb 9.9 g/dl which was normochromic and normocytic but his reticulocyte count was twice normal. He had a normal total white count but a low lymphocyte count ($0.8 \times 10^9/l$) and his platelet count was normal. Urea and electrolytes and liver function tests were normal. His ANA was strongly positive to titre 1:5,120 with a speckled pattern. Anti-Sm antibody was detected but he had no antibodies to DNA and his C3 was normal. His Coombs test was strongly positive but he had no anti-phospholipid antibodies.

Questions

1 Describe the abnormality seen in the figure.
2 What additional antibody test has shown to be very useful in distinguishing RA from SLE?
3 Is surgery advised to correct the hand deformities?
4 How useful is the anti-Sm antibody in making a diagnosis of lupus?
5 How common is a severe, Coombs' positive anaemia in patients with lupus?

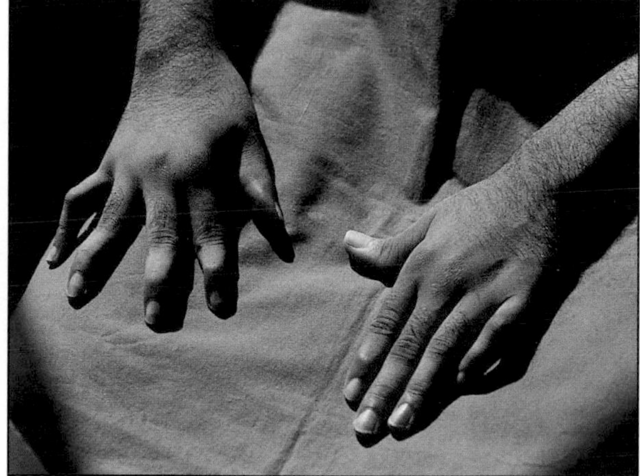
45

CASE 46

A 30-year-old woman was diagnosed with polyarticular juvenile idiopathic arthritis (JIA) at the age of 7 years. Her disease persisted into adulthood. At her routine follow-up appointment she expressed a desire to become pregnant. Her medication at that time included leflunomide 20 mg/day and methotrexate 15 mg/week.

Questions

1 What advice would you give about the patient's medication?
2 Does JIA affect her fertility?

CASE 45

Answers

1 The figure shows the typical appearances of Jaccoud's arthropathy. Essentially this is due to hypermobility, causing subluxation of the meto-carpophalangeal joints, proximal interphalangeal joints and distal interphalangeal joints. There is no true synovitis and on x-ray erosions are rarely seen. Jaccoud's is seen in fewer than 5% of patients with lupus.

2 In contrast to IgM rheumatoid factor, present in the majority of patients with RA and a significant minority of lupus patients, anti-CCP antibodies have been found to be virtually diagnostic of RA, very rarely occurring in other conditions.

3 Provided the patient's hands remain functionally effective surgery is not advised. Although it may achieve a more normal looking hand, functionally the results are disappointing.

4 The presence of anti-Sm antibodies are a diagnostic criterion for lupus although only detectable in around 10% of Caucasian lupus patients and 35% of Afro-Caribbean patients.

5 Coombs' positivity is present in around 20% of lupus patients, but Coombs' positive haemolytic anaemia causing an Hb of less than 10 g/dl is present in fewer than 5% of patients.

CASE 46

Answers

1 Both drugs need to be stopped. The active metabolites of leflunomide have been shown to be teratogenic. The manufacturers advise leaving 2 years between stopping the drug and conception. It is possible to reduce this time by 'washing out' with cholestyramine or active charcoal. Either way, levels of the active metabolite should be less than 20 μg/l in two blood samples, taken 14 days apart, before conception is considered safe. Methotrexate is also teratogenic. There is no washout option with this drug, but a gap of at least 3 months should be left between stopping methotrexate and attempting to conceive. Although steroids do have some potential harmful effects, they are considered the safest option during pregnancy. Azathioprine can also be used to try to keep the steroid dose down.

2 JIA does not directly affect fertility. It can however have a deleterious effect on pelvic development and can make vaginal delivery impossible.

CASE 47

A 60-year-old man presented with a history that over several years he had noticed painful swelling and stiffening of several proximal (PIP) and distal interphalangeal (DIP) joints. He volunteered that the pain in each joint eventually settled but that each remained stiff and swollen. He also had pain when gripping at the base of his right thumb. His father had had a similar problem. He was hypertensive and taking diuretic and a calcium channel blocking agent. His blood results are shown in *Table 47*.

The x-ray of his hands is shown (47).

Table 47 Blood test results

Hb	12.8 g/dl
WBC	7.2 x 10^9/l
Plt	250 x 10^9/l
ESR	22 mm/h
CRP	<5 mg/l
RF	1:40
Urate	530 μmol/l

Questions

1 What does the x-ray show?
2 What is the most likely diagnosis?
3 What is the differential diagnosis?
4 How should the patient be managed?

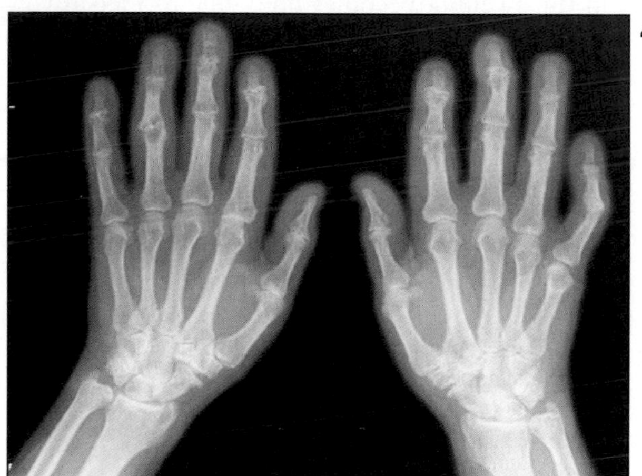

47

CASE 48

A 27-year-old woman was brought to the emergency department by her boyfriend. He was concerned because for the preceding 3 days she had been behaving oddly. He described her as usually shy in nature, but she had been acting as though she were drunk, being excitable and aggressive. A diagnosis of systemic lupus erythematosus (SLE) had been made 2 years earlier, when she had been referred to a rheumatologist with a facial rash, hair loss, arthritis and a strongly positive ANA. A week before this admission, she had been started on 40 mg prednisolone for a flare of her arthritis, with instructions to reduce the dose over 7 days. She was referred to the medical team because there was some concern that the bizarre behaviour might represent neurological involvement of her SLE. She had an MRI brain which was normal, and a lumbar puncture. This showed an opening pressure of 8 cm, glucose 4.0 mmol/l (serum glucose 5.0 mmol/l), protein 0.3 g/l, no WBC and no RBC.

Questions

1 What is the differential diagnosis?
2 What other tests would you do to clarify the most likely diagnosis?

CASE 47

Answers

1 There is loss of joint space of several DIP and PIP joints and the first carpometacarpal (CMC) joints. There are also osteophytes around the affected joints.

2 The history is typical of nodal osteoarthritis which is often familial. Typically each joint becomes swollen, red and painful, often one at a time. The pain and redness settle usually over several months and the swelling becomes bony due to Heberden's nodes (DIPs) and/or Bouchard's nodes (PIPs). This is often associated with pain and stiffness at the base of the thumb, eventually leading to adduction of the thumb metacarpal bone.

3 The rheumatoid factor is at low titre and although the picture can be confusing if the DIPs are not affected and the PIPs swollen, rheumatoid arthritis is unlikely in the absence of other joints being affected. Although the urate is raised because he is on a diuretic, this is not a typical history of gout and the urate level can be ignored.

4 Explanation and reassurance that the problem rarely causes long-term disability is helpful. Involvement of the PIPs causes finger stiffness and is undoubtedly more disabling than when the DIPs alone are affected. There is no evidence yet that the problem can be stopped or reversed. Some try local NSAID gels, a low cholesterol diet or glucosamine with chondroitin but there is little evidence that they affect the natural history. If a joint is acutely inflamed it can be treated by injection of a small volume of a corticosteroid which will settle the acute pain but again does not affect the long-term outcome. Occasionally the advice of an expert hand surgeon should be sought.

Outcome

The patient was reassured. He tried glucosamine and chondroitin for 3 months but was not persuaded it helped and gave up. He managed quite well despite the stiff fingers but eventually went to see a hand surgeon about an unstable index finger DIP which was fused in slight flexion. He decided against surgery for his still painful right CMC joint.

CASE 48

Answers

1 Cerebral lupus can present in this way, even in the absence of abnormalities in the CSF or on imaging. The main differential would be steroid-induced psychosis.

2 In order to differentiate between the two, it is helpful to look for ongoing disease activity in other organs. Rising titres of DNA antibodies or falling complement, or evidence of active lupus in the kidneys such as worsening proteinuria or red cell casts would suggest that the personality change was from the disease itself. Conversely, no evidence of disease elsewhere, accompanied by improving blood tests, would favour steroid-induced psychosis.

CASE 49

A 57-year-old Pakistani woman with Sjögren's syndrome, Raynaud's syndrome, depression and hypothyroidism presented with a 10-month history of profound fatigue, muscle ache and weakness affecting the thighs and arms. She noticed difficulty climbing stairs and getting off a low chair; she could hardly grip her handbag or comb her hair. In addition, she complained of intermittent watery diarrhoea for the last 5 months, mild left iliac fossa pain and weight loss of 3 kg in 4 months. There was no history of skin rash, night sweats or fever. A colonoscopy showed some diverticular disease and biopsies were normal. Blood tests are shown in *Table 49*.

Questions

Part A

1 In light of her persistent muscle weakness, what additional investigations are indicated?

Part B

The patient underwent a muscle biopsy. The histology was reported as showing '... mononuclear cell invasion of non-necrotic muscle fibres, vacuolated fibres. Intracellular amyloid deposits were identified by fluorescent method.'

2 What is the diagnosis?
3 What is the aetiology and prognosis of this condition?
4 What are the treatment options?

Table 49 Blood test results

Hb	12.5 g/dl	IgA	2.1 g/l
WBC	8.4 x 10^9/l	IgG	25.4 g/l
Plt	320 x 10^9/l	IgM	2.6 g/l
Glucose	Normal	C3	Normal
Magnesium	Normal	C4	Normal
Calcium	Normal	ESR	70 mm/h
Phosphate	Normal	RF	1:320
Vitamin D	Normal	ANA	1:1280
Cortisol	Normal	DNA antibodies	10 IU/ml
TSH	Normal	Anti-Ro antibody	Positive
Free thyroxine	Normal	Anti-La antibody	Positive

CASE 50

A 67-year-old woman with long-standing ankylosing spondylitis (AS) fell 4 feet off a ladder. She immediately developed upper thoracic back pain which got worse over the next 24 hours when she presented to her local emergency department. The lateral x-ray of her cervical spine is shown (50a).

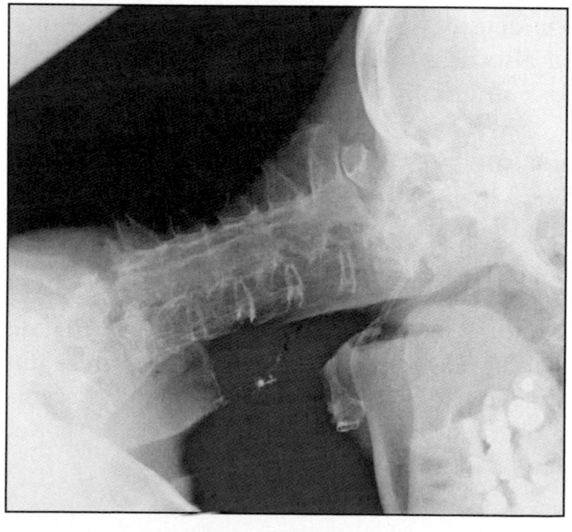

50a

Questions

1 What does the x-ray show?
2 How should the patient be managed?

CASE 49

Answers

1 Further investigation would comprise: myositis antibodies testing including anti-Jo-1, muscle enzymes (CK, LDH), malignancy screen including tumour markers, myeloma screen, EMG, MRI muscles, muscle biopsy, liver function tests, abdomen and pelvic imaging and chest x-ray.
2 Sporadic inclusion body myositis (S-IBM). Note the vacuolated muscle fibres and mononuclear invasion of non-necrotic muscle fibres. If electron microscopy also shows 15–18 nm tubulofilaments or amyloid deposits then these findings confirm the diagnosis.
3 The aetiology is unknown. S-IBM presents both inflammatory and degenerative features. It has been likened to a prion disease, but some theories suggest that muscle damage may also be the consequence of a primary T cell-mediated autoimmune response.

The prognosis is poor and in many cases the muscle weakness slowly progresses.
4 The disease is resistant to steroids, several immunosuppressives and empiric treatments. Interferon beta-1a, high dose vitamin C, carnitine, coenzyme Q10, mycophenolate mofetil, IV immunoglobulin and prednisolone, anti-thymocyte globulin and methotrexate have been tried with varying success. Studies are underway involving the use of agents such as etanercept, lithium and the T cell depleting monoclonal antibody, alemtuzumab.

CASE 50

Answers

1 There is an unstable fracture through the pedicles at C6/7, with angulation and involvement of the three columns. There are also changes compatible with longstanding AS – fusion of the spine (bamboo spine) and apparent osteopenia.
2 This is a neurosurgical emergency. Immediately, the patient should have immobilization of the spine and full neurological assessment, which was normal. Further imaging with a CT confirmed the findings. She underwent a C7 corpectomy with case and plate fusion, and a C5–T2 posterior fusion. The postsurgery x-ray is shown (**50b**). Fortunately, she made a complete recovery, with no neurological sequelae. In the longer term, she requires assessment of bone density and appropriate management. She should also be advised to be very careful to avoid high risk situations!

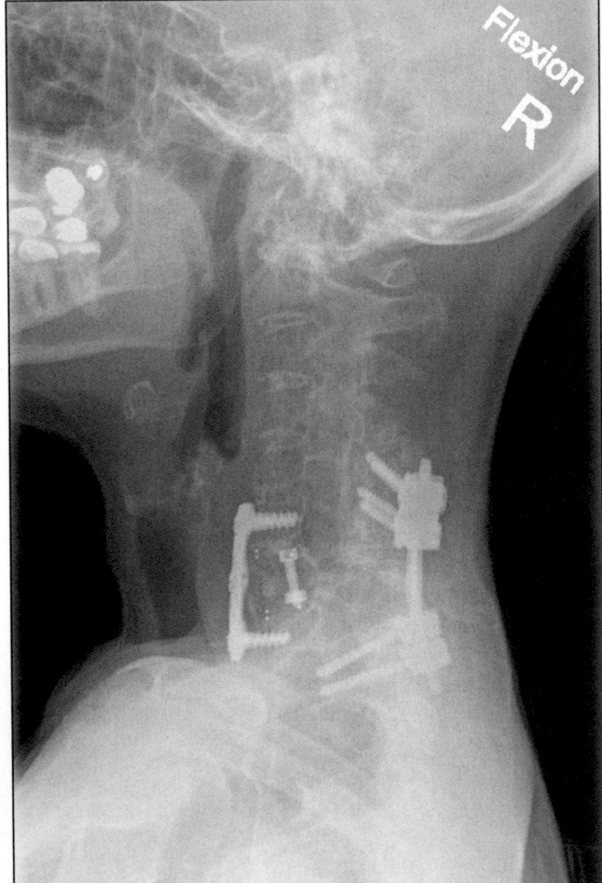

50b

Discussion: Fractures in AS

Patients with AS are at increased risk of fracture, particularly in the spine. This is partly because of an increased risk of osteoporosis, and partly because of reduced spinal flexibility. In addition, they have long-standing back pain and consequently often do not present until relatively late because they put up with the pain. It is important to make patients aware of fracture risk, and insist they present after any significant trauma.

CASE 51

A 24-year-old woman noticed that over a 2-month period she was finding it increasingly difficult to rise from the squatting position in her gym. Subsequently she found that lifting heavy books off an office shelf just above where she sat at her desk was becoming more difficult.

She went for a holiday to Ibiza during the summer and towards the end of her stay she noticed a striking rash on her forearms and hands (**51**). On her return she went to see her primary care physician who noted grade 4/4+ proximal muscle weakness in her arms and legs as well as the associated rash. There was no family history of muscle weakness, no other major previous medical history or other relevant history. The primary care physician referred her to the local rheumatology department where the primary care physician's findings were confirmed and investigations were performed (*Table 51*).

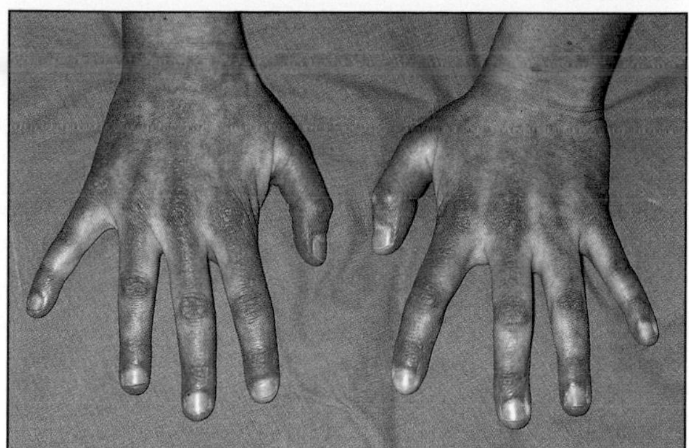

51

An EMG showed multiple small polyphasic low amplitude potentials typical of a myopathic pattern. Muscle needle biopsy of the patient's left quadriceps was undertaken but was reported to be normal.

Table 51 Results of investigations

Hb	12.7 g/dl
WBC	6.3 x 10^9/l
Plt	380 x 10^9/l
ALT	97 IU/l
CK	3,218 IU/l

Questions

1 What is the rash, and the overall diagnosis, and is this a typical distribution?
2 Is the raised ALT confirmatory of an associated autoimmune liver disease?
3 Is the CK in the typical range for patients presenting in this way?
4 Does the normal muscle biopsy question the diagnosis?
5 What is the role of corticosteroids in the treatment?

CASE 52

A 46-year-old woman of African descent was seen in a university clinic with a history of malar rash, photosensitive rash, polyarticular inflammatory arthritis, seizure disorder, deep venous thrombus in both legs and pulmonary embolus. Laboratory investigations included a positive ANA at 1:3,240, anti-dsDNA by *Crithidia luciliae* assay at 1:270, anti-cardiolipin antibodies positive at 26 GPL, anti-Sm and anti-RNP positive by ouchterlony. There was additionally a several-year history of pemphigus, currently flaring with widespread, painful, deep, blistering lesions, unresponsive to prednisone and azathioprine.

The patient was started on the following combination therapy: mycophenolate 1 g/day, azathioprine 150 mg/day, hydroxychloroquine 200 mg bd and prednisone 40 mg/day. Over the course of the next several weeks, the lesions began to resolve.

Questions

1 What is the association between lupus and pemphigus?
2 How might this affect treatment?

CASE 51

ANSWERS

1 The rash of dermatomyositis is, as shown in the figure, typically on the extensor surfaces of the forearms and hands.

2 It seems likely that some so-called 'liver enzymes' may in fact be made in skeletal muscle, and these are often raised in patients with myositis. Often the AST is more elevated than the ALT.

3 Yes, the CK in patients presenting with acute dermatomyositis is often between 1,000 and 5,000 IU/l.

4 The Bohan and Peter (1975) criteria confirm that three out of the following criteria make a diagnosis of myositis: history of proximal muscle weakness, raised CK enzyme, myopathic EMG and typical changes in myositis on a biopsy. Myositis may, rarely, be a strikingly focal disease and it seems probable in this case that the muscle needle biopsy simply missed an affected area.

5 Although corticosteroids are invariably used (starting doses in the region of 0.5 mg/kg in the acute phases of this disease are often used) there is no definitive double blind trial evidence to support their efficacy.

CASE 52

ANSWERS

1 Lupus can be a risk factor for pemphigus foliaceus, which is a relatively superficial lesion, characterized by burning or itching blisters on the scalp, face, neck, armpits or trunk, or pemphigus vulgaris, which extends to deeper layers of the skin and may also involve the mouth and mucous membranes. Pemphigus erythematosus (Senear–Usher syndrome) represents a crossover lesion which resembles pemphigus foliaceus, and can be found in patients with lupus. Lesions tend to be relatively restricted to the malar eminence, mantle region and upper back, not extending down the trunk. Bullae are common or erythematous plaques with vesicles, erosions or scale. Direct immunofluorescence usually detects immunoglobulin and complement in the epidermis or at the dermal–epidermal junction, similar to a lupus lesion.

2 The mainstay of treatment for all forms of pemphigus is steroids and immunosuppressants. It may be necessary, as in this case, to try several regimens before optimal therapy is derived. It is important to watch the progress of a patient like this carefully, since, if allowed to progress, pemphigus can be life threatening.

CASE 53

A fit 70-year-old tennis player presented with a sudden history of severe and swelling behind and below the medial malleolus while playing tennis. At the same time he noticed that his foot has suddenly become much flatter. He had had flat feet all of his life. There was a 4-week history of less severe pain with swelling in the same place. On examination the foot was flat (pronated) and there was marked tenderness and swelling behind and below the medial malleolus. He was unable to stand on the toes of this foot or to evert the ankle. The subtalar joint felt unstable. There was no swelling of the ankle joint.

Questions

1 What is the most likely reason for the patient's foot suddenly going flat?
2 What is the best investigation to demonstrate the cause?
3 What might have been done if the patient had presented earlier?
4 How should the patient be treated?

CASE 54

A 55-year-old banker was referred because of pain in both hands. The pain had come on gradually over the preceding 12 months. His hands were stiff in the mornings, and he felt he had become clumsy. The pain was worst in the evenings, especially after spending a lot of time at the computer. In addition, he complained of worsening fatigue. He was not taking any medication.

On examination he had bony swelling over the second and third metacarpophalangeal joints bilaterally. The joints were not hot or red, but were slightly tender. He was unable to extend fully the index and middle fingers of both hands. X-rays of his hands are shown (54). Blood tests are shown in *Table 54*.

54

LT R

(Courtesy of Hussain *et al.* [2010] *Rapid Review of Radiology*, CRC Press.)

Questions

1 What is the diagnosis?
2 How would you confirm this?
3 How should the patient be managed?

Table 54 Blood test results

Hb	15.9 g/dl
WBC	7.6×10^9/l
Neutrophils	3.2×10^9/l
Plt	305×10^9/l
Albumin	38 g/l
ALT	187 IU/l
Bilirubin	14 μmol/l
ALP	98 IU/l
Urea	6.0 mmol/l
Creat	98 μmol/l
ESR	12 mm/h
CRP	6 mg/l
RF	Negative
Anti-CCP	Negative

CASE 53

ANSWERS

1 He has almost certainly torn the tendon of the tibialis posterior muscle. This stabilizes the hind foot against eversion. The differential diagnosis of medial ankle pain is most commonly a sprain of the deltoid ligament and other medial ankle structures following an eversion injury, a fracture of the medial malleolus or occasionally a stress fracture or avascular necrosis of the navicular bone. None of these would lead to the suddenly flattening of the foot. A fracture of the medial malleolus would produce tenderness over the malleolus rather than posterior and below it.

2 Ultrasound is the best way of finding the cause although it will also be seen on an MRI scan. The tendon can be visualized along its length and in the tarsal tunnel – under the flexor retinaculum which retains the tibialis posterior tendon and the tendon of flexor hallucis longus as they round the medial malleolus.

3 Chronic tibialis posterior tenosynovitis is relatively common and more likely in people who are active and have flat feet, whether rigid (developmental) or flexible (hypermobility in the young, or ageing). The swelling and tenderness may be marked and extend to the medial arch. There may be associated tarsal tunnel syndrome – pain, tingling and numbness of the medial ankle and on the sole of the foot, particularly at night. This is due to compressing of the posterior tibial nerve in the tarsal tunnel. Assuming that there was no partial tear of the tendon or significant longitudinal splitting of the tendon (tendonosis) on ultrasound at the time when there was pain and swelling, a local corticosteroid injection into the tendon sheath would have helped. When combined with a medial arch support it might have reduced the risk of a complete tear. With a significant tendonosis it is probably best to avoid a corticosteroid injection and put the foot in a resting lightweight cast in inversion and plantar flexion for about 3–6 weeks.

4 At the age of 70 years it may not be possible to repair the tendon permanently although as the patient is still physically active a specialist foot surgical opinion should be sought. In the short term the pain can be reduced by using a resting cast or a removable Aircast® ankle splint with a fitted medial arch support. Unless it can be repaired, the foot will remain flat and the patient will be dependent on arch supports.

Outcome

Ultrasound showed a full tear of the tendon just below the medial malleolus. There was no fracture on x-ray. The patient went ahead to have a surgical repair but this failed. He continues to play tennis, but less vigorously with a moulded arch support and high-sided sports shoes.

CASE 54

ANSWERS

1 Haemochromatosis.

2 Elevated serum ferritin is the next screening test (>200 μg/l males, >100 μg/l females), with an elevated transferring saturation: serum iron/TIBC >45%. Thereafter patients go on to have haemochromatosis gene (HFE) typing, and a liver biopsy done if cirrhosis is suspected.

3 Phlebotomy does not help arthropathy, but usually it responds to NSAIDs. Some patients require arthroplasty.

CASE 55

An 80-year-old Italian man presented to his optician with a 1-month history of a red eye (55). The eye seemed to have become a little protuberant and on questioning it was associated with some nasal stuffiness and a troublesome left sided headache. He was also troubled by some polyarthralgia with genuine swelling at the wrists which had developed about the same time as his red eye.

Apart from several fractures (he had worked as a builder and a roofer), there was little of note in his previous medical history. There was similarly little of concern in his family history, and apart from 'steroids' for mild asthma no drug history of relevance.

He was treated with steroid eye drops which improved his eye temporarily but the problem flared again about a month later and his joint pain and swelling were becoming worse. He was referred to the local rheumatology unit where baseline investigations showed a normal Hb and WBC and differential, but an ESR of 97 mm/h and a CRP of 56 mg/l, a negative ANA and rheumatoid factor of 1:40.

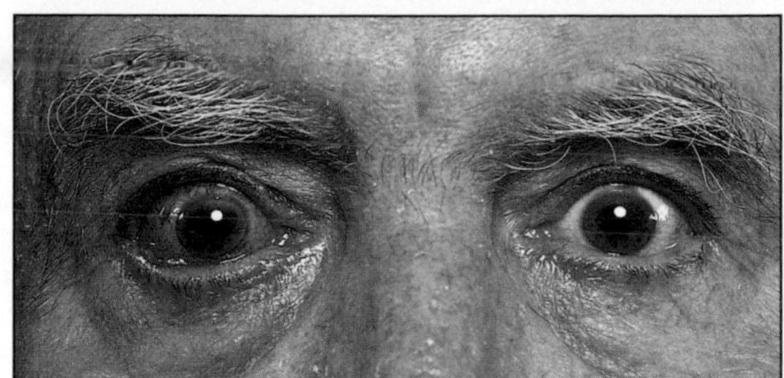
55

Questions

1 What other autoantibody should be sought, what is its precise target and what is the frequency in the disease with which it is most closely associated?
2 What is the most likely diagnosis in this case?
3 What are the organs and systems most commonly involved in this condition?
4 Suggest an initial treatment programme for this patient.
5 What is the approximate mortality associated with this disease?

CASE 56

A 39-year-old Caucasian accountant was admitted with a history of right sided headache, dizziness, photophobia and transient deafness. Examination revealed no ophthalmoplegia or other cranial nerve signs. His fundus was normal. Blood pressure was 150/82 mmHg. Blood tests revealed ESR of 38 mm/h and CRP of 19 mg/l. Haemoglobin, platelet count and WBC count (including differential) were normal. A CT head and lumbar puncture were normal. Four weeks later he presented ahead of a planned outpatient clinic review with a history of fever, aches in the calves, thighs and upper arms. He also complained of night sweats, tenderness over the maxillary sinuses and difficulty hearing from the right ear. He denied any chest pain, urinary symptoms, abdominal pain, diarrhoea or constipation.

In his past medical history, he had a single attack of uveitis 9 years ago. He suffered from hayfever and mild asthma and had been prescribed loratidine tablets and beclomethasone and salbutamol inhalers for this.

Clinical examination revealed proximal weakness in the upper and lower limbs, bilateral symmetrical sensory deficit affecting the medial border of the soles of both feet and depressed reflexes in the upper and lower limbs. A few scattered wheezes were heard in his chest.

Repeat blood tests revealed CRP of 113 mg/l, ESR of 62 mm/h, CK of 389 IU/l; 24-hour creatinine, protein and calcium were normal. HbA1c, thyroid function tests, bone profile and electrolytes returned normal. His urea was slightly elevated at 8.0 mmol/l with a creatinine of 87 μmol/l. Liver function tests were normal. FBC revealed low Hb of 10.8 g/dl, platelet count of 427 × 10^9/l and WBC count of 14.40 × 10^9/l. The eosinophil count was elevated.

Questions

1 What is the likely condition?
2 What additional aspects of the patient's history should be asked about?
3 What further investigations might be required?
4 Are there risk factors which predict a worse outcome in some patients with these conditions?

CASE 55

Answers

1 Antibodies to anti-neutrophil cytoplasmic antigens (ANCA) should be measured. The precise target is serine proteinase 3 and antibodies to this target are found in approximately 85% of patients with granulomatosis with polyangiitis (GPA) (formerly Wegener's granulomatosis).

2 GPA is indicated.

3 It is a multisystem disease, with often widespread pathology. The most commonly involved organs/systems are the ear, nose and throat, kidney, lungs, eye, heart, skin, musculoskeletal and nervous systems.

4 Traditionally, a combination of oral corticosteroids and cyclophosphamide are used. Prednisolone is often started at 1 mg/kg/day for up to 3 months, tapering over the next 12 months to approximately 0.2 mg/kg/day. Cyclophosphamide can be given as an oral regimen starting with 2 mg/kg/day or as IV pulses monthly for several months. Maintenance regimens usually include a combination of prednisolone and azathioprine. More recently, B cell depletion with rituximab has also been used as induction therapy.

5 Untreated, mortality is 90% at 2 years. Treated, mortality varies, with estimates reported from 14% to 56% at 10 years.

CASE 56

Answers

1 This is a vasculitis and features so far are most suggestive of eosinophilic granulomatosis with polyangiitis (EGPA) (formerly Churg–Strauss syndrome).

2 The patient should be asked about history of use of recreational intravenous drugs, sexual history, travel history, immunization history, history of testicular pain (common in polyarteritis nodosa) and family history.

3 Workup for a vasculitis can be extensive and may include screening for autoimmune conditions, infection and malignancies. Any or all of the following may be indicated: autoimmune profile including ANA, ANCA, rheumatoid factor, dsDNA, extractable nuclear antigen, anti-cardiolipin antibodies and lupus anticoagulant, serum ACE, serology for hepatitis C and B, HIV, TB and other mycobacteria, parvovirus B19, cytomegalovirus, herpes zoster, urinalysis for active urinary sediment (casts and RBC), cryoglobulins, blood cultures, stool examination for parasites, fungal cultures, cultures of mucosal surfaces, EMG/nerve conduction studies, audiogram, gallium scan, biopsy of skin, kidney, muscle or nerve, imaging of sinuses, chest, abdomen and pelvis, echocardiogram, ECG and angiography.

4 The five-factor score was developed in 1996 by the French Vasculitis Group for EGPA and polyarteritis nodosa and has subsequently been validated for microscopic polyangiitis. A score of 1 point is assigned for each of the following: proteinuria > 1 g/24 h, creatininaemia > 140 µmol/l, specific gastrointestinal involvement, specific cardiomyopathy and specific CNS involvement. The lower the score the higher the 5-year survival. Five-year survival falls to 54.1% with scores of 2 or above.

Outcome

The patient was found to have negative anti-neutrophil cytoplasmic antibodies but raised IgE levels and peripheral blood eosinophilia >10% with negative toxicology and stool screen for parasites. A biopsy of the left deltoid revealed vasculitic lesions of the intermuscular blood vessels with infiltration of eosinophils in and around the blood vessels. Sinus CT scan revealed a pansinusitis. Chest x-ray showed interlobular septal lines. He was diagnosed as having EGPA. Initial treatment was commenced with high dose prednisolone (1.0 mg/kg/day) to which he made a good response with resolution of fever, chest, sinus muscle and neurological symptoms. At follow-up 4 weeks later, he had no symptoms but was not keen to persist with oral prednisolone at tapering doses as he was very concerned about possible side-effects. He was started on oral azathioprine 2.0 mg/kg/day but suffered a severe relapse of chest and muscle symptoms at 5 months requiring pulses of IV methylprednisolone for 3 days.

CASE 57

A 15-year-old girl presented with a 1-month history of an intermittent rash on her trunk, and a lesion on her left elbow (57). Three days prior to presentation she developed synovitis affecting the small joints of her hands. She felt generally unwell, and had a low grade fever. Investigations are shown in *Table 57*.

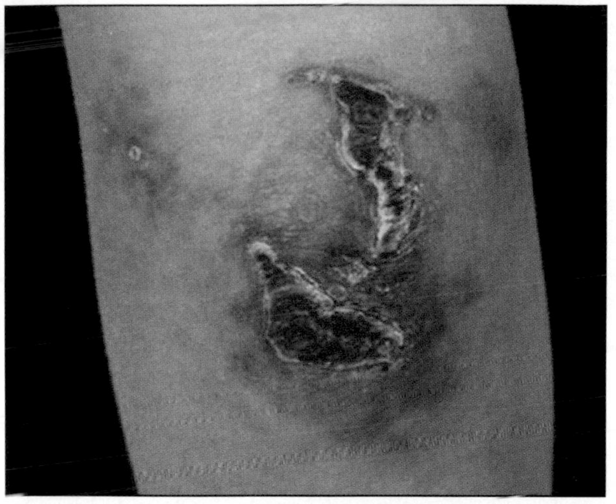

57

Questions

1 What is the most likely diagnosis, and the key differentials?
2 What additional investigations are required?
3 How should this patient be treated?

Table 57 Results of investigations

Hb	10.2 g/dl	CK	150 IU/l
WBC	5.0 × 10^9/l	Urea	6.0 mmol/
Plt	400 × 10^9/l	Creat	64 μmol/l
Albumin	32 g/l	ESR	12 mm/h
ALT	60 IU/l	CRP	6 mg/l
AST	93 IU/l	RF	Negative
Bilirubin	14 μmol/l	Anti-CCP	Negative
ALP	98 IU/l	ANA	Negative
LDH	200 IU/l	ANCA	Negative

CASE 58

A 42-year-old man presented with pain in the right groin. He had been limping noticeably for several months. He was a weekend footballer and otherwise fit and well. He did not recall any sporting injury. On examination he had reduced rotation in flexion of the right hip and a fixed flexion deformity of about 10°. An x-ray of his hip was taken (58).

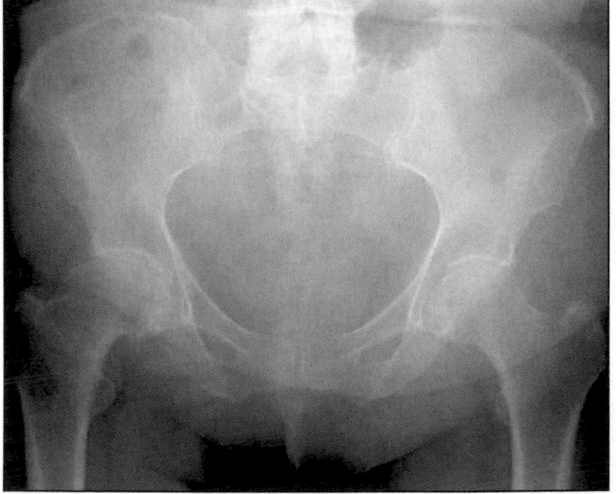

58

Questions

1 What does the x-ray show?
2 What is the differential diagnosis of groin pain in a sportsperson?
3 How would you manage this patient?

CASE 57

ANSWERS

1 Juvenile dermatomyositis (JDM). The ulcerated lesion over the left elbow is a feature of JDM that may be more obvious than the classic rashes such as a heliotrope rash over the eyes or Gottron's papules over the metacarpophalangeal/proximal interphalangeal joints. The differential diagnosis would include systemic lupus erythematosus, and a small vessel vasculitis, although these are made less likely by the absence of positive antibodies. CK can be normal or only marginally elevated. However, muscle damage is also indicated by the elevated AST and LDH.

2 EMG is not usually done in children. MRI is used to localize affected muscle, and guided biopsy confirms the diagnosis.

3 In view of the ulceration, treatment with high dose IV steroids was started, and she subsequently received a course of IV cyclophosphamide. In milder cases, oral steroids with a steroid-sparing agent such as methotrexate or azathioprine may suffice.

Discussion: JDM and malignancy

Unlike in the adult form of the disease, JDM is not associated with an increased risk of underlying malignancy; however, in this case as the age was borderline, screening was considered appropriate.

CASE 58

ANSWERS

1 There is osteoarthritis (OA) of the hip. This is unusual in a patient of this age and is associated here with acetabular dysplasia. The shallow acetabulum places increased stress on its lateral margin and on the acetabular labrum and this appears to be the reason for the early development of OA. Sometimes patients present with hip pain due to acetabular dysplasia but without OA. In the young patient there is then justification for referral to an expert hip surgeon to review the need for a preventative acetabular osteotomy.

2 OA of the hip is unusual at this age without a precipitating cause such as Perthes' disease, avascular necrosis (in a diver for example) or sickle cell disease. The restricted movement on examination and the fixed flexion deformity are highly suggestive of hip disease in this case. Much more common are injuries of the soft tissues in the groin. This includes adductor tendonosis or enthesitis, psoas bursitis or injury to the insertion of the rectus femoris into the superior pubic ramus. These can be readily seen on MRI, which is the diagnostic method of choice if simple measures such as rest and analgesia do not help.

3 The patient will be distressed by the diagnosis and may not yet want to consider surgery or even a surgical referral. It is worth seeing if analgesics or NSAIDs will help to maintain normal activity. It is best that he gives up football but keeps fit and maintains a low weight with low impact (cross trainer) or non-weight bearing exercise (cycling). A review with a new x-ray in 3–6 months will then permit an assessment and will probably demonstrate to the patient that seeing an orthopaedic surgeon is best. He will need a hip resurfacing procedure, with reconstruction of the acetabulum. Total hip replacement is now avoided at this age and up to the age of 65 years when possible.

Outcome

The patient was sufficiently disabled that he wanted to see an orthopaedic surgeon. They both decided to wait 6 months but analgesia was not helpful and he went ahead to surgery. Five years later he is active and pain free but no longer plays football.

CASE 59

A 63-year-old woman noticed that her eyes were becoming increasingly irritable when trying to put in her contact lenses and that when eating dry biscuits or crackers she seemed increasingly to require a glass of water at the same time. Accompanying these problems, which developed over a period of 7 months, she became severely fatigued and noted a pain without swelling in her hands and feet and some lack of concentration.

She discussed the problems with her primary care physician who reassured her that this was 'just getting old' and prescribed her an antidepressant, which simply made her mouth even more dry. Eventually while visiting her dentist, who was most concerned at the increasing amount of dental caries, it was suggested that she might attend a local rheumatology clinic known to have an interest in this sort of problem.

On questioning in the clinic she also admitted that she increasingly disliked bright lights and that her eyes were rather itchy. There was nothing of relevance in her previous medical history but in her family she mentioned she had a cousin with an underactive thyroid gland.

On examination the appearance of her lips (59) was striking. An absence of a salivary pool beneath the tongue was noted and the eyes were a little red. There was no lymphadenopathy and her pulse, blood pressure and heart sounds were normal, as was examination of her respiratory system, abdomen and CNS. Examination of the locomotor system revealed Heberden's nodes in several fingers but no evidence of synovitis.

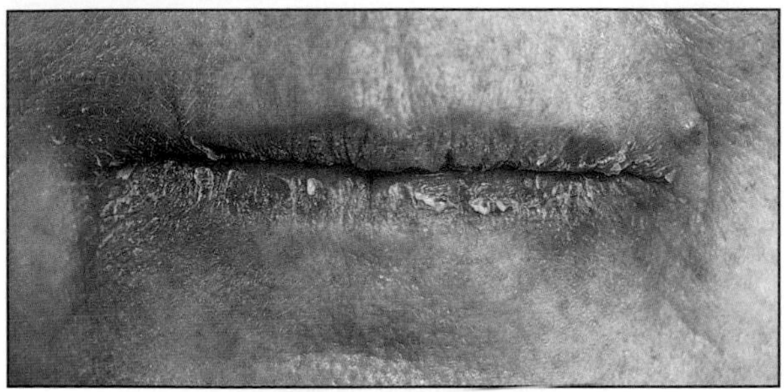

59

A Schirmer's test showed damping of the test strips to less than 5 mm to both eyes. Among the blood tests undertaken her Hb was 14.2 g/dl, normal white count and platelets, urea and electrolytes and liver function test were normal. ANA was positive to a titre of 1:2,560 as were antibodies to Ro and La. Her ESR was 57 mm/h and total IgG was 30 g/l (normal = 8–18). Electrophoretic strip showed no evidence of any individual paraprotein.

QUESTIONS

1 Is this patient's age against the diagnosis of Sjögren's syndrome?
2 What neurological complications are well known to be associated with Sjögren's?
3 Is high IgG an uncommon feature of Sjögren's and does it suggest an underlying malignancy?
4 At what frequency are autoantibodies seen in Sjögren's syndrome?
5 Will this patient benefit from a low dose of corticosteroids?

CASE 60

This 32-year-old man presented to the emergency department with stridor and type 1 respiratory failure (60). He had a normal chest x-ray and his autoantibodies were all negative. His blood count was normal, but his ESR was 42 mm/h and his CRP 28 mg/l.

QUESTIONS

1 Describe the abnormal findings in **Figure 60**.
2 What additional information would you try to elicit from the history?
3 What is the differential, and the most likely diagnosis in this patient?
4 How should the patient be managed?

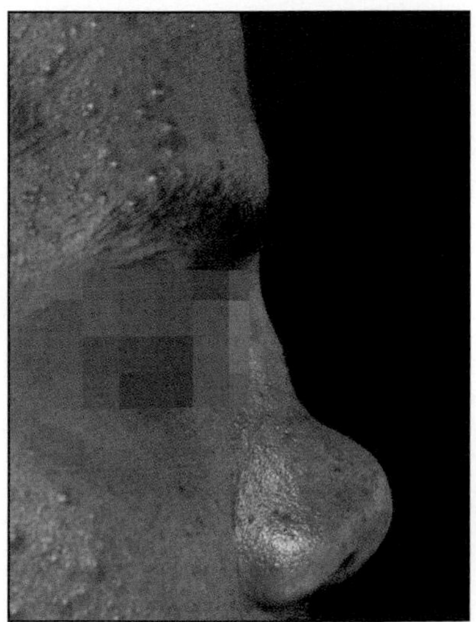

60

CASE 59

Answers

1 The majority of patients present between the ages of 50 and 70 years. It is, in contrast, a very rare disease in patients under the age of 20 years.
2 Periphery neuropathy, carpal tunnel syndrome and trigeminal neuralgia are the best recognized neurological complications of Sjögren's. More serious neurological events occur in fewer than 5% of Sjögren's patients.
3 The hypergammaglobulinaemia seen in this patient is typical of many patients with primary Sjögren's syndrome (the IgG level is often higher in Sjögren's patients than in lupus patients) and this is not an undue cause for concern about an underlying malignancy.
4 Anti-nuclear antibodies are present in 80–90% of patients with Sjögren's syndrome, usually with a speckle pattern and often in association with anti-Ro (60–80%) and anti-La (30–40%); rheumatoid factor is also present in 50–60% of these patients.
5 There is no evidence that steroids in high or low doses are of value in treatment of patients with Sjögren's syndrome.

CASE 60

Answers

1 Collapsed bridge of the nose. Papular rash on the face.
2 The patient should be asked about the onset of his collapsed nose bridge; episodes of ear pain; the onset of the rash; and if there are symptoms of nasal crusting/bleeding.
3 GPA is unlikely given negative anti-nuclear cytoplasmic antibodies and normal chest x-ray; and congenital syphilis would only account for the collapsed bridge of the nose. Relapsing polychondritis (RP) is the most likely diagnosis in this case.
4 Management of RP is mainly based on case series at best. Given severity with respiratory failure the patient needs high dose corticosteroids, and additional immunosuppression. In milder forms, azathioprine or methotrexate is used. In this case, the patient was treated with IV cyclophosphamide for 6 months then switched to azathioprine after remission was induced. He required a tracheostomy because of tracheomalacia, a well recognized and dangerous complication of RP.

CASE 61

A 55-year-old woman presented with a 3-week history of pain in the right forefoot. It was highly localized and worse when weight bearing. On examination there was swelling and she was tender over the fourth metatarsal bone. She was well otherwise. X-ray of the foot is shown (**61a**).

QUESTIONS

1 What is the diagnosis?
2 How should the patient be investigated?
3 What is the differential diagnosis of forefoot pain?
4 What is the treatment?

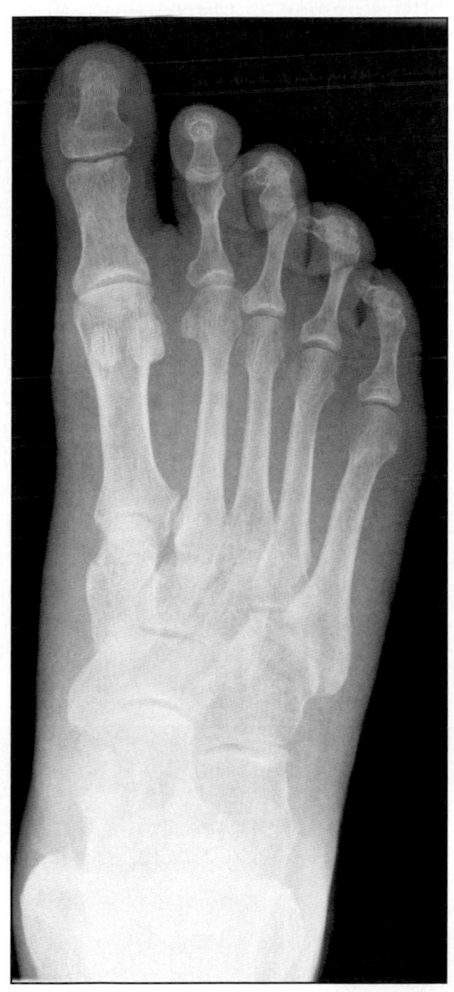

61a

CASE 61

ANSWERS

1 The most likely diagnosis is a stress (march) fracture. This often does not show up immediately on x-ray, as in this case.

2 If the diagnosis is unclear the fracture will show up readily on an isotope bone scan although it may be simplest to x-ray again in 3 weeks if the pain persists. The differential diagnosis of persistent forefoot pain is best sorted out by MRI scanning. The patient is menopausal so it is wise to check for risk factors for osteoporosis:

- early menopause without hormone replacement,
- a family history of osteoporosis (for examples fractures or loss of height in her mother),
- a personal history of little exercise, a calcium poor diet, amenorrhoea (sports or eating disorder), heavy smoking or alcohol intake, or the use of steroids.

A dual energy x-ray absorptiometry (DEXA) scan is worth considering.

Figures 61b and **61c** show the plain film and MRI of another example, with a healed fracture.

3 Simple metatarsalgia causes pain in the ball of the foot and may be due to unaccustomed walking or thin soled shoes. Trainer-type shoes will help. A Morton's neuroma causes pain at the base of two adjacent toes (usually third and fourth or second and third) and painful 'pins and needles' on the apposed sides of the affected toes. Bursitis between two metatarsal heads may produce similar symptoms. MRI scan will demonstrate these and they can be treated by a local steroid injection by a rheumatologist or under x-ray guidance. Metatarsalgia is very common in rheumatoid arthritis and occasionally is the presenting symptom. Osteoarthritis of the great toe metatarsophalangeal joint produces pain and stiffness (hallux rigidus) of the joint. Gout produces severe pain, swelling and redness usually of the great toe but may be associated with gouty cellulitis of the foot.

4 For a stress fracture supportive shoes with thick soles and reduced walking usually suffice.

Outcome

The pain settled over 6 weeks with trainers and rest. The patient was a professional ballet dancer during earlier years and had amenorrhoea for 10 years. Her mother had fractured a hip. She had a DEXA scan with T score (comparison with ideal bone density at age 30 years) of –3.0 in the lumbar spine and –2.8 in the left hip and was diagnosed as osteoporotic. She was started on bisphosphonates and calcium with vitamin D3 and given dietary and exercise advice. Her bone density increased to the osteopenic range after 1 year and stabilized. (Osteopenia T = –1 to –2.5. Osteoporosis T = < –2.5.)

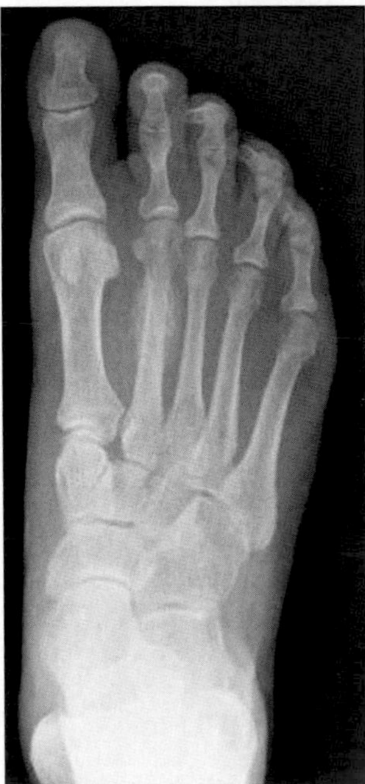

61b

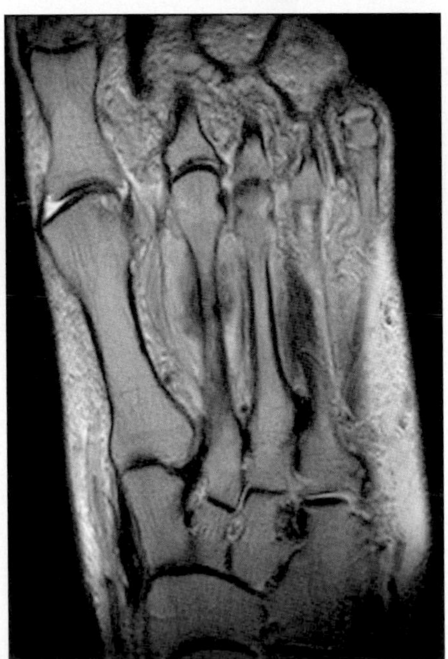

61c

CASE 62

A 59-year-old woman was referred by her primary care physician with a recurrent, intermittent rash on her shins, feet, buttocks and arms. The lesions were round, raised and red, were initially itchy, but then became painful. One of the lumps had come to a head and leaked a white, creamy discharge. The scars from a previous episode in the preceding year were still visible on her shins. With the onset of the rash the patient described fever, arthralgia and right upper quadrant pain. Her chest x-ray was normal. The rash on her lower legs and feet is shown (**62a, 62b**).

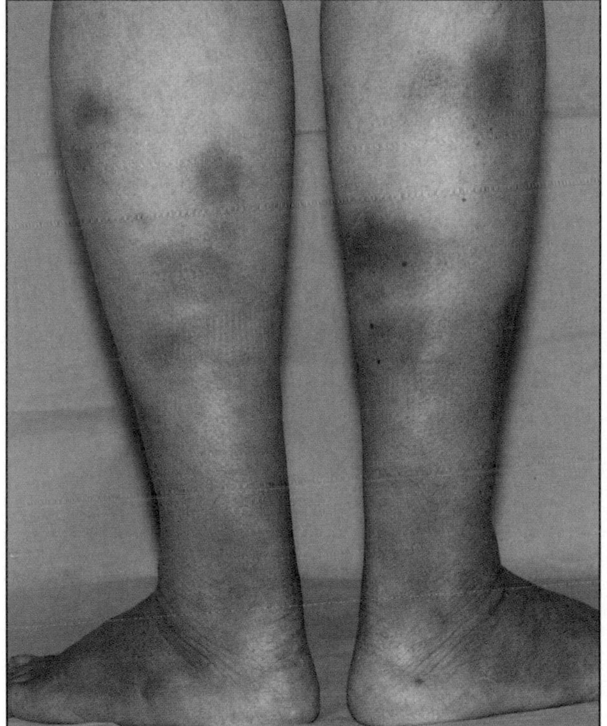

62a

Questions

1 What is the differential diagnosis of these lesions?
2 What is the most likely diagnosis in this case and which investigations would you request to confirm your diagnosis?

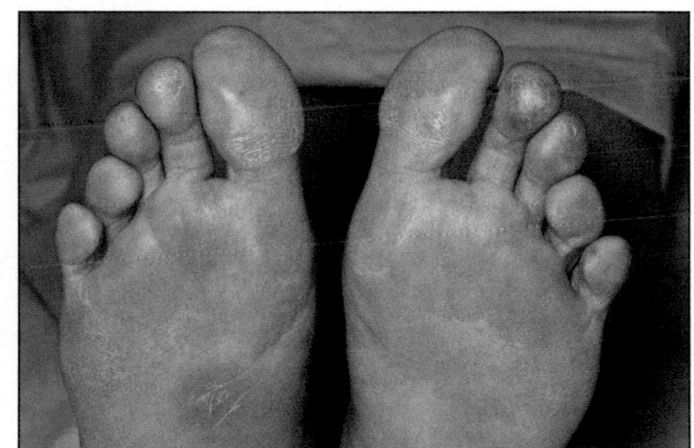

62b

CASE 63

A young man presented with a 5-day history of severe shoulder pain. There had been no injury although he played a lot of sport. The pain limited all movements of the shoulder and was predominantly felt in the region of the deltoid. He was otherwise well. His shoulder x-ray is shown (**63**).

Questions

1 What does the x-ray show?
2 What is the differential diagnosis of shoulder pain and restriction in a young person?
3 What complication might arise in this patient?
4 How would you treat him?

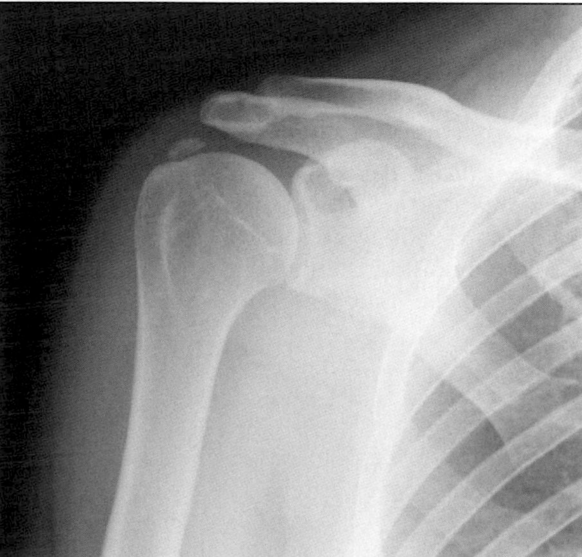

63

CASE 62

Answers

1 The lesions are typical of panniculitis, defined as inflammation of the subcutaneous tissue. The most common form of panniculitis is erythema nodosum (EN), but in this case there are particular features which suggest an alternative diagnosis. EN is usually confined to the shins and rarely affects the trunk or arms. The lesions of EN classically heal without scarring, and do not suppurate.

The differential diagnosis of panniculitis is broad, and the association of the symptom with arthralgia and fever suggest the need to exclude systemic lupus erythematosus. Other diseases to be considered include inflammatory bowel disease, pancreatitis, α-1-antitrypsin deficiency, lymphoma, sarcoidosis and TB.

2 In this particular case, the patient was diagnosed with pancreatic panniculitis. She was investigated with a skin biopsy and CT abdomen. The skin biopsy must be deep enough to include the subcutaneous tissue, and confirmed lobular panniculitis. Her CT abdomen revealed gallstones. Although by the time of her outpatient visit her serum amylase was normal, her lipase was found to be elevated. A presumptive diagnosis of gallstone pancreatitis was made.

CASE 63

Answers

1 There is a calcific deposit in the supraspinatus tendon. This is unusually large and the calcification is often difficult to see but usually lies just proximal to the insertion of the tendon into the greater tuberosity of the humerus.

2 More commonly in such cases the x-rays are normal and the diagnosis can only be made by ultrasound examination when there may be a tendonosis of the rotator cuff, usually of supraspinatus. There may be a complete or partial tear of the affected tendon. There may also be an associated or isolated subacromial bursitis. The severe restriction of movement here was due to the severity of the pain but may suggest an inflammatory arthritis or a developing adhesive capsulitis of the shoulder. The short history is against either of these diagnoses.

3 The calcific deposit may break through into the bursa causing an acute calcific bursitis. This is seen as a cloudy appearance on x-ray between the acromion and the humerus. The pain is often severe and the joint feels hot and is swollen. The differential diagnosis is of septic bursitis only if there is no cloudiness on x-ray.

4 The best approach would be to inject the subacromial bursa with 40 mg methylprednisolone acetate or 20 mg triamcinolone acetate or hexacetonide, using local anaesthetic to insert the needle from the side, just below the acromion. The patient will need high doses of an oral NSAID such as naproxen 500 mg bd with food. If this fails, ultrasound guided breaking up of the deposit with a needle under local anaesthetic (barbotage) followed by steroid is best but may worsen the pain initially by causing a calcific bursitis. Occasionally the deposit is removed surgically.

Outcome

The patient did not respond to the initial injection but recovered rapidly once the deposit was broken up under ultrasound guidance. He made a full recovery. The reason for such deposits forming is not known.

CASE 64

A 33-year-old man presented with a 3-week history of severe left knee pain and swelling. He had a swollen great toe on the right foot. He did not recall an injury. He felt unwell but had not been feverish. There was no recent history of joint problems but he was unwell with vomiting and diarrhoea a couple of weeks before the joints became painful, and became dehydrated, but had recovered without treatment. He had not been abroad. There was no known family history to help. He had taken a few ibuprofen tablets.

On examination the knee was warm, inflamed and swollen with an effusion. It was painful to move and had a slight fixed flexion deformity. It flexed to about 100°. The great toe was diffusely swollen and red. There was nothing else to find on examination. Results of blood tests are shown in *Table 64*. Liver and renal function were normal.

Table 64 Blood test results

Hb	12.0 g/dl
WBC	10.3 x 10^9/l
Neutrophils	8.0 x 10^9/l
ESR	63 mm/h
CRP	55 mg/l

Questions
1 What is your differential diagnosis in this case on the information given?
2 What is the most likely diagnosis?
3 What one further investigation would you choose?
4 How would you treat this patient?

CASE 65

The 42-year-old man whose thoracic spine x-ray (65) is shown below had psoriatic arthritis and was being treated with methotrexate and etanercept.

He presented with a 6-week history of well localized back pain which had worsened significantly in the past week. He found it difficult to walk down the stairs because of the pain. There was no history of trauma to the spine. The patient complained of profound fatigue, night sweats and weight loss of 3 kg. In the past week he had developed a low grade fever. His pain and fever had failed to respond to ibuprofen and paracetamol in maximum doses.

Questions
1 What is the key finding on the x-ray?
2 What is the most likely cause of this finding?
3 List important differential diagnoses.

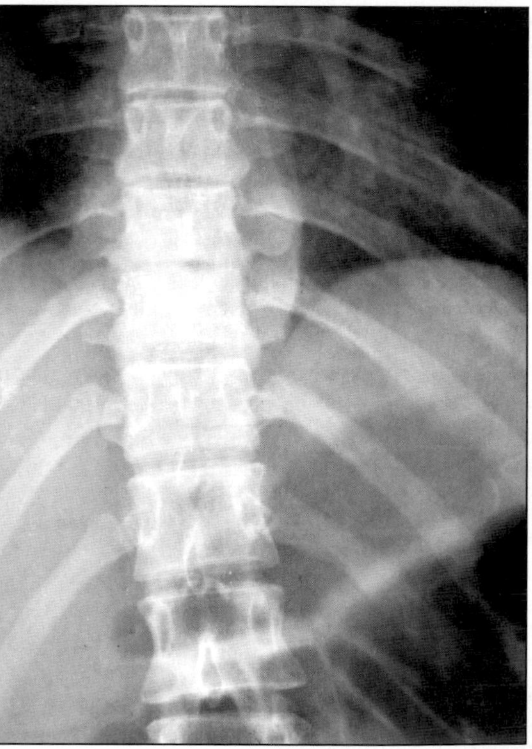
65

CASE 64

Answers

1 The recent history of diarrhoea and vomiting is the most important clue and suggests a reactive arthritis, probably to *Salmonella* spp. The swollen 'sausage' toe with diffuse swelling is also typical of a seronegative spondyloarthropathy. There may be a personal or family history of psoriasis, chronic inflammatory bowel disease or inflammatory back pain, worse in the morning suggesting sacroiliitis and ankylosing spondylitis. Although the patient is young and there is no known family history, gout is possible. The great toe metatarsophalangeal joint is usually affected and is agonizing at onset. There may be an associated gouty cellulitis which often extends onto the dorsum of the foot. Polyarticular gout is unusual but can occur. The dehydration would have been relevant if more recent as this can precipitate gout. Even when not fully treated with adequate doses of NSAIDs, the typical gouty attack settles in about 7–14 days, making this diagnosis less likely in this patient's case.

Injury may cause acute knee pain due to a torn meniscus which causes immediate swelling, and tenderness on the medial or lateral side of the knee. The joint is not usually warm or hot to the touch unless there is a haemarthrosis, for example associated with a torn anterior cruciate ligament. In such circumstances the injury is always significant and would not have been forgotten. It is usually so painful that the individual presents to the emergency department.

Rheumatoid arthritis may present as a monoarthritis of the knee but this is less common. Women are affected more often than men.

Septic polyarthritis in an otherwise fit man is usually associated with fever and malaise, so unlikely in this case. The only proviso is if he were immunosuppressed due to undiagnosed HIV infection when the systemic symptoms may be muted.

2 The most likely diagnosis is reactive arthritis after a bacterial dysentery (either *Salmonella* spp. or *Shigella* spp., occasionally *Yersinia* spp.).

3 Aspiration of the joint would be important and if you are unable to do it, the patient should be referred urgently for a rheumatology opinion. Examine the fluid – and send it for urgent Gram staining and culture, and polarized light microscopy.

4 If confident that the fluid is not infected and the patient not septic, consider injecting the joint with 20–40 mg triamcinolone hexacetonide or 40–80 mg methylprednisolone acetate followed by 24 hours relative non-weight bearing and give oral NSAIDs in full doses. (If you feel this is a septic arthritis, treat with oral NSAIDs until culture results are obtained and refer as a medical emergency and for admission. Microbiological advice should be sought.) Some patients with reactive arthritis require a short oral course of prednisolone to settle things. If the arthritis persists, although this is unusual, the patient needs specialist care and will probably need either sulphasalazine or methotrexate.

Outcome

The fluid was cloudy but not purulent so 80 mg methylprednisolone acetate was injected and the patient was given diclofenac slow release 75 mg bd. The fluid was negative for organisms on Gram stain and culture and no crystals were seen. The diagnosis was of reactive arthritis. He required a short course of oral steroids and remained on NSAIDs for 3 months but made a full recovery. There was no point treating with antibiotics as the infection had cleared several weeks before he presented. He did not require sulphasalazine or methotrexate.

CASE 65

Answers

1 The x-ray shows a paraspinal abscess.

2 TB is the most likely cause.

3 The differential diagnosis includes subacute infection due to other organisms such as *Staphylococcus aureus* and atypical fungal infection.

CASE 66

A 47-year-old woman was referred to the rheumatology clinic complaining of widespread joint pain, intermittent diarrhoea and weakness and fatigue. This had become progressively worse over the preceding 6 months. Examination revealed normal joints. There was mild weakness of hip flexion, but otherwise neurological examination was also normal. Blood tests showed normal full white cell and platelet count, but Hb was 10.9 g/dl, with a normal mean cell volume, but a red cell distribution width of 18%. Renal function and CK were normal. ALP was elevated at 180 IU/l, and vitamin D low at 22 nmol/l, but calcium and phosphate were normal, as were bilirubin and ALT. ESR and CRP were within normal limits.

Questions

1 What further tests would you request?
2 What is the diagnosis, and how should the patient be managed?

CASE 67

A man aged 53 years was seen in a rheumatology department complaining of difficulty in rising from a chair, running upstairs and playing his usual 18 holes of golf. He had no skin rash and apart from a little shortness of breath, thought likely to be due to a concomitant history of asthma, he had no other clinical features. There was nothing of note in his previous medical history but he did smoke 20 cigarettes a day and he drank a bottle of wine every 2–3 days.

On examination, he looked well and there was no lymphadenopathy. However, some expiratory wheezing was heard in his chest though his pulse, blood pressure and heart sounds were normal. Examination of his nervous system revealed grade 4+ weakness in his quadriceps but there was no other weakness and his reflexes were all intact.

Investigation included a slightly raised ESR at 30 mm/h, normal Hb, WBC and platelets. In addition his urea and electrolytes were normal. His ALT was elevated at 90 IU/l (normal <45) and his CK was 2,412 IU/l (normal <190). His EMG showed myopathic changes and the muscle biopsy confirmed the presence of an inflammatory myopathy.

He was treated with prednisolone and azathioprine, very successfully, for 1 year but as the dose of these drugs was reduced his proximal weakness began to return. In addition, for the first time, he began to complain of some distal weakness in his left leg. He found it very difficult, for example, to rise on tiptoe on the left side. An MRI scan was obtained (67).

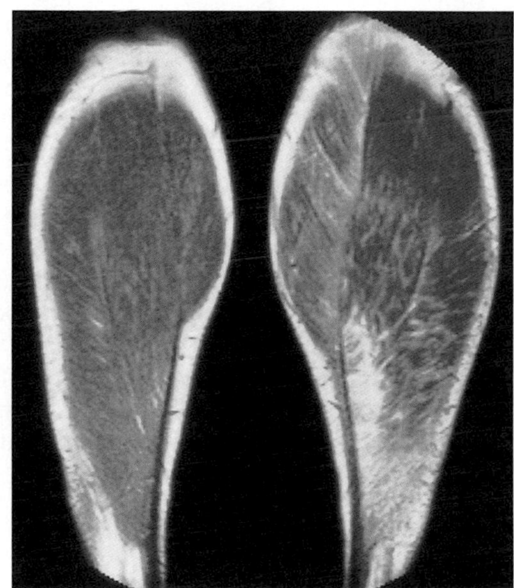
67

Questions

1 Is myositis found as commonly in men as in women?
2 This patient's ANA was positive to a titre of 1:320 but his Jo-1 antibody was negative. Is this strong evidence against the diagnosis of myositis?
3 Jo-1 is a tRNA synthetase enzyme (for each of the 20 amino acids there is one unique accompanying enzyme). How many of these enzymes have shown to be targets in patients with myositis?
4 Given that the combination of steroids and azathioprine was not effective, what combination might you choose next to treat his autoimmune muscle disease?
5 What does the MRI show?

CASE 66

ANSWERS

1 Available bloods suggest malabsorption; further blood tests should include: iron, B12, folate, anti-endomysial and anti-gliadin antibodies, plus an endoscopy with duodenal biopsies to confirm the diagnosis histologically.

2 The features of this case indicate coeliac disease. The patient requires a gluten-free diet, and additional vitamin D and iron/folate/B12 supplements.

CASE 67

ANSWERS

1 Myositis is seen in women two to three times more commonly than in men.

2 Antibodies to Jo-1 are found in approximately 25% of patients with myositis only, i.e. the majority of patients with myositis do not have antibodies to this enzyme.

3 Eight of the 20 synthetase enzymes have been identified as targets in patients with myositis; these are histidyl (Jo-1), threonyl (PL7), alanyl (PL12), isoleucyl (OJ), glycyl (EJ), asparingyl (HS), tyrosyl (ARS) and phenylalanyl (Zo). In all, approximately 30% of patients with myositis have antibodies to these synthetase enzymes.

4 If steroids and azathioprine are not effective most rheumatologists would switch to steroids and methotrexate. Occasionally a combination of steroids and methotrexate and IV immunoglobulin, given every 3 months for up to a year, can be very effective.

5 The MRI scan in the T2 weighted image shows increased swelling and whiteness compatible with inflammation. Weakness in the distal muscle, gastrocnemius, of his left leg was unexpected and unusual and so biopsy was repeated. This confirmed the rather unusual inflammatory change in the unilateral distal muscle.

NB. It is important to remember to investigate for underlying malignancy. Although more common in dermatomyositis, it is also associated with polymyositis.

CASE 68

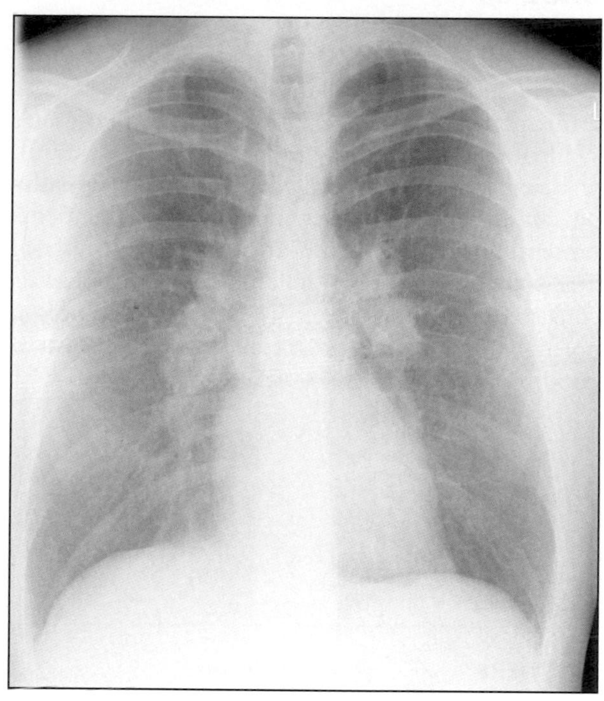
68

A 34-year-old housewife came to the clinic complaining of sudden onset of painful swelling affecting her lower legs, which had started 2 weeks earlier. Initially, she had noticed pain in both shins, which she thought was shin splints as she was a keen runner, but a week later she noticed swelling and pain in both ankles. Usually an active person, she felt tired and complained of fevers up to 37.7°C. On examination, there were tender lumps overlying both shins, and marked synovitis of both ankles. In addition, a painless enlarged lymph node was found in the cervical chain.

Blood tests were as follows – FBC normal, ESR 32 mm/h, CRP 25 mg/l, renal/liver/bone profiles all normal and serum ACE normal. Multiple blood cultures and a throat swab were sterile. ASO titres were normal. She had had a BCG, and a Mantoux test was anergic. A chest x-ray was taken (**68**).

Questions

1 What is the differential diagnosis?
2 How should she be investigated further?

CASE 69

A 35-year-old woman of mixed Caucasian and Native American descent was at 31 weeks' gestation when she suddenly developed a photosensitive rash on her face and upper chest, followed by fevers, chills, hair loss, arthritis of the fingers, wrists, elbows, knees and ankles, painful mouth sores that prevented eating, muscle aches and shortness of breath. She was treated for 4 weeks with low dose prednisone without relief before presenting to a university prenatal care centre. On examination she appeared acutely ill, with a prominent subacute cutaneous-like rash, shallow palate ulcers, tender proximal muscles and synovitis of multiple joints. Laboratory tests were notable for a leucocyte count of 3,000/μl, Hb 8.5 gd/l, absolute lymphocytes of 276/μl and an active urinary sediment with haematuria and 3+ protein. ANA was positive at 1:1,080, anti-dsDNA by *Crithidia* assay was positive at a titre of 1:7,290. Complement components C3 and C4 were low.

The patient was treated with 1 mg/kg prednisone and rapidly improved. The baby was delivered near term without complications. Subsequently a renal biopsy was performed, with a finding of mesangio-proliferative nephritis with low activity and chronicity scores. The patient was treated with prednisone for 4 months and azathioprine for 9 months until she developed severe hair loss. During this period she was virtually asymptomatic with normal urinalysis and protein as well as decrease in anti-dsDNA titre to 1:90. Hypocomplementaemia persisted.

She remained well for an additional 2 years on hydroxychloroquine 200 mg PO bd. Review of systems was negative for signs or symptoms of illness. Laboratory studies were unremarkable except for a rise in anti-dsDNA to 1:270 and persistent hypocomplementaemia. There had been no return of rash, systemic illness or arthritis and no evidence of active nephritis.

Questions

1 After an explosive onset of systemic lupus, how common is it for a patient to have completely quiescent disease for several years?
2 How would pregnancy be expected to play a role?
3 What evidence is there that monitoring of this patient should continue?

CASE 68

Answers

1 The most likely diagnosis is acute sarcoid arthropathy. The classical presentation of Lofgren's syndrome is the triad of erythema nodosum (EN), ankle or knee arthritis and bihilar lymphadenopathy on chest x-ray. However, up to 10% of patients presenting with an acute arthritis have a normal x-ray. The low grade inflammatory response is consistent with the diagnosis. Serum ACE is often normal in the acute presentation, and suggests a good prognosis.

2 Other possibilities include TB and lymphoma. In view of the enlarged cervical lymph node which is slightly atypical, biopsy should be performed to confirm the diagnosis. Other possible biopsy sites include the lip or hilar lymph nodes. A gallium scan may show typical 'sarcoid' features, and may demonstrate evidence of disease elsewhere.

Discussion

Acute sarcoid arthritis usually responds to NSAIDs. Occasionally patients require more therapy such as oral steroids.

CASE 69

Answers

1 This is an atypical case. Onset of lupus, particularly nephritis, during pregnancy is associated with poor fetal outcome and it is rare for the disease to remain quiescent for several years, given the moderate treatments that this patient received.

2 Patients with pre-existing lupus may flare during pregnancy but the literature does not support increased risk for flares during this time. Pregnancies in lupus patients are high risk due to the potential for several complications, including miscarriage, fetal growth retardation, premature birth, pre-eclampsia/eclampsia, the HELLP syndrome and neonatal lupus syndrome, which in rare cases can result in complete heart block in the infant.

3 The persistence of antibodies to dsDNA and low complement, which are associated with lupus flares, suggests the need to continue monitoring this patient. Notably the original high titre of anti-dsDNA by the *Crithidia* assay was the highest titre ever recorded in that laboratory.

CASE 70

A 45-year-old woman had had pain in the upper arm for about 3 months. Initially she was able to move the arm but found it painful at about 90° of abduction and she could not do up her bra. The pain was worse at night. It had worsened gradually and was now severe and she was unable to move the shoulder even to wash under her arm. She was sleeping badly because of the pain and was disabled by the stiffness. She had been well and the only past history was of a similar episode of pain in the other shoulder a few years ago for which inexplicably she did not seek any treatment – it lasted about 18 months. Her blood test results are presented in *Table 70*. Her liver and renal function were normal for her age.

The x-ray of her shoulder is shown (70).

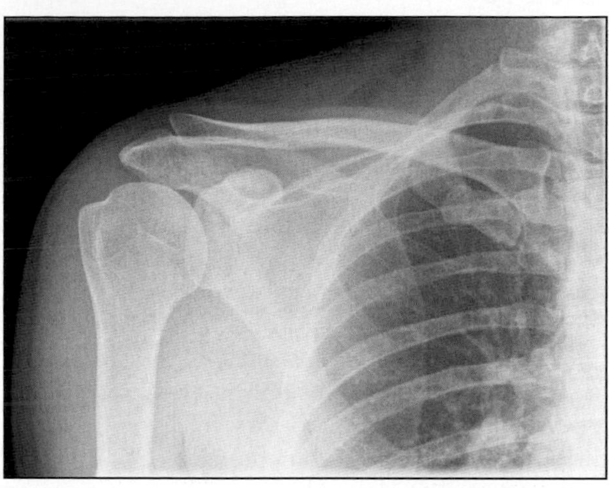
70

Table 70 Blood test results

Hb	12.5 g/dl
WBC	9.00 x 10^9/l
Neutrophils	6.10 x 10^9/l
ESR	15 mm/h
CRP	<5 mg/l

Questions

1 What is the diagnosis if you had seen the patient before the shoulder stiffened?
2 How would you have treated her then?
3 What is the diagnosis now?
4 How should the patient be treated?

CASE 71

Figures 71a and **71b** show pictures of a 19-year-old girl's hands and scalp, respectively.

Questions

1 What do these pictures show?
2 What are the cutaneous complications?

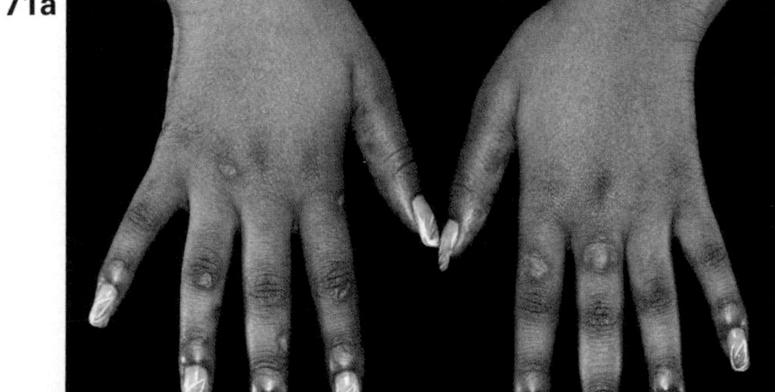
71a

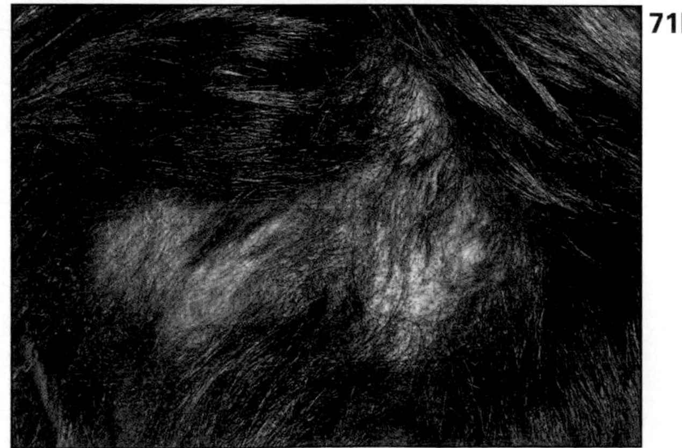
71b

CASE 70

Answers

1 The patient presents the typical features of a rotator cuff tendonosis with pain in the upper arm, worse on abduction (a painful arc) and keeping her awake at night.

2 The pain can be helped by sedative analgesia at night and NSAIDs, but the quickest way to relieve the pain is to inject steroid subacromially. This is a straightforward procedure which can be undertaken in the clinic as long as aseptic technique is scrupulous. It is not usually necessary to do an x-ray at this stage unless the first injection fails. The differential diagnosis was a complete or partial tear of the affected tendon. There may be an associated or isolated subacromial bursitis. This is best demonstrated by a diagnostic ultrasound procedure undertaken by an expert. The treatment for all is the same, although some caution needs to be exercised if there is a significant tear as an injection may in theory worsen it.

3 The severe loss of all movements suggests that the patient has developed an adhesive capsulitis (true frozen shoulder). The aetiology is unclear. X-ray and MRI if undertaken are usually normal. An acute monoarthritis is less likely in this case because the blood tests are normal.

4 This is a difficult problem to treat. In the initial painful and stiff stage there is some evidence that serial injections of steroids into the joint and subacromially speed up pain relief. Hydrodilatation, using a larger volume of local anaesthetic and steroid, is favoured by some and may be more effective. Usually the patient requires strong analgesia and NSAIDs as well. Once the painful phase has settled, usually after about 3 months, stiffness remains and lasts up to 12 months. During the stiff phase there is some evidence that either subacromial release or a manipulation under anaesthetic speeds recovery of the movement; although this may never be complete, it is rarely disabling in the long term. It may recur as it had in this patient.

Outcome

The pain remained very troublesome despite three sets of injections and strong analgesia for about 4 months, then gradually resolved. The patient opted to avoid surgery and recovered 90% of the range of movement over the next year.

CASE 71

Answers

1 Discoid lupus.

2 Scarring alopecia and infection.

CASE 72

A 30-year-old woman presented to the emergency department with a gradually worsening pain over the dorsum of the foot and up the front of the shin. She had noticed that the top of the foot was swollen. She did not recall an injury but was training for a half marathon. On examination there was swelling from the mid point of the dorsum to the ankle. There was crepitus when she moved her toes over the same area and in the shin. The ankle was not swollen.

Questions

1 What is the cause of the swelling and the crepitus?
2 What treatment would you suggest? – she still wants to continue training!
3 What is the differential diagnosis of dorsal foot and anterior ankle pain?

CASE 73

A 63-year-old woman was started on etanercept and methotrexate for seropositive rheumatoid arthritis. Seven months into the treatment she presented to the emergency department with a rash on her hands and feet (**73a, 73b**).

Questions

1 What is the rash?
2 What is the cause?
3 How should her arthritis be managed now?

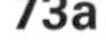
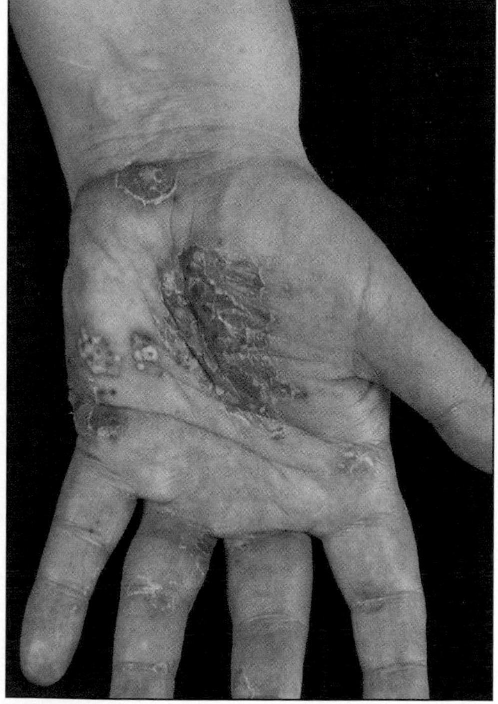
73a

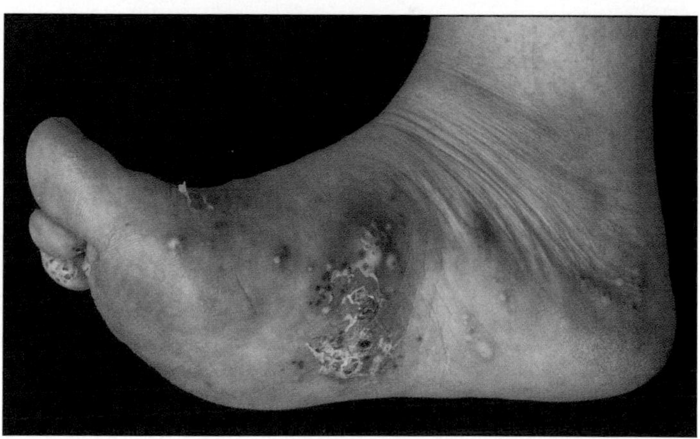
73b

CASE 72

Answers

1 The description is typical of dorsal or extensor tenosynovitis of the foot, which can be brought on by unaccustomed walking or exercise or sometimes by tight shoes. The tendon sheath is swollen. The extensor hallucis and tibialis anterior tendons pass under the extensor retinaculum and also under a retaining ligament over the lower tibia. It is the inflammation that causes this crepitus. The muscles are in the upper anterior compartment of the lower leg.

2 She will need to rest for a while and be patient. Binding the foot and lower leg with the ankle in a neutral position helps, but recovery will be speeded by the insertion of a corticosteroid injection into the extensor tendon sheath. She must rest for a few days after the injection and then go back gradually to exercise. Good running shoes with a medial arch support and not too tight lacing will help prevent a recurrence.

3 Pain in the mid foot may be due to a stress fracture; this is more common in osteoporosis. There is local pain, swelling and tenderness over the affected metatarsal bone. The fracture can be demonstrated on a plain x-ray but may not be immediately visible. A bone scan or MRI at the early stage is diagnostic. Mid tarsal pain in an older patient may be due to mid foot osteoarthritis. In inflammatory arthritis of the ankle the swelling and pain are around the ankle.

Outcome

Although not keen, the patient stopped training, had an injection of 25 mg hydrocortisone acetate, wore an elastic bandage from below the knee to the mid foot when walking for about 3 weeks and then returned gradually to exercise. She bought new running shoes and completed the half marathon the next year.

CASE 73

Answers

1 Palmar–plantar pustular psoriasis.

2 It has been triggered by the use of a TNF inhibitor – etanercept – an uncommon but recognized side-effect of treatment. This is intriguing given TNF inhibition is also used for the treatment of psoriasis and associated arthritis.

3 The etanercept must be stopped. This is not considered a class effect so alternative TNF inhibitors can be used, but it has been associated with all the drugs. Alternatively, a switch to an alternative biologic such as rituximab could be considered. There are very few case reports of pustulosis triggered by rituximab. As the patient was very distressed by the rash, she was switched to rituximab.

CASE 74

A 64-year-old man developed a left leg deep vein thrombosis (DVT) after a 22-hour flight and was commenced on warfarin tablets. He had a 3-month history of untreated hyperlipidaemia with a low HDL cholesterol, and a 10-year history of gout for which he had been taking allopurinol 100 mg od. When advised by the pharmacist that allopurinol could potentiate the effect of warfarin, he promptly discontinued allopurinol.

Three days later, his knees became grossly swollen, red and painful. His primary care physician commenced colchicine 500 µg bd on suspicion of a gouty flare. After 2 days, he had diarrhoea and refused to take any more colchicine. His ankles subsequently became swollen and he could not weight bear. He was admitted to hospital.

His INR was 1.8, CRP 68 mg/l, ESR 49 mm/h, WBC 11.0 × 10^9/l, neutrophils 75%, serum urate 7.0 µmol/l, urea 4.3 mmol/l and creatinine 82 µmol/l on admission. X-rays of both knees showed minor osteoarthritic changes. The knees were aspirated and the findings at microscopy of the synovial fluid from the left knee are shown (**74**). No organisms were detected on Gram stain.

Question

How should the patient be managed?

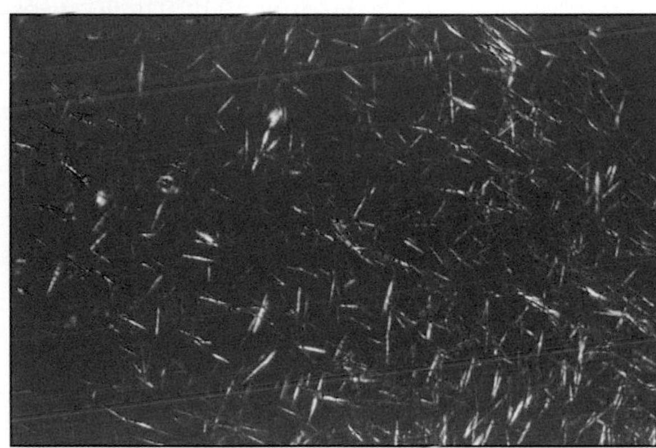

74

CASE 75

Figure 75 shows the hands of a 23-year-old woman.

Questions

1 What does the figure show?
2 What is the differential diagnosis?

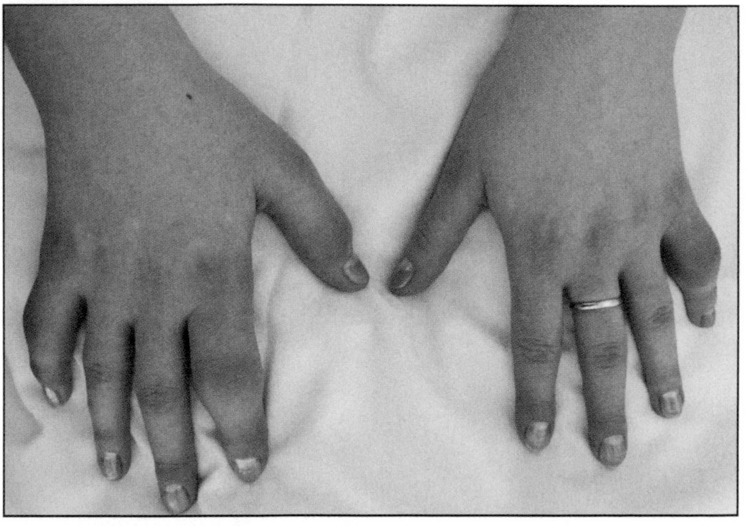

75

CASE 74

Answer

Allopurinol should not be restarted during an acute flare of gout. Some practitioners will not give intramuscular steroids, or perform intra-articular injections unless the INR is less than 1.5 to reduce the risk of haematoma or intra-articular bleeds. He could be prescribed a short course of oral steroids, e.g. prednisolone 25 mg od, tapering the dose as he improves to the lowest possible maintenance dose to control symptoms. Appropriate bone protectants and a proton pump inhibitor should be prescribed. Low dose NSAIDS should be used with caution in view of warfarin.

Once the joint swelling subsides, gentle physiotherapy should be commenced. Since this patient is not mobilizing much, his warfarin treatment should be optimized to keep the INR between 2.0 and 3.0. DVT treatment is usually for 3–6 months. When the patient is off warfarin then allopurinol may be restarted under colchicine or steroid cover. Alternatively, he may be prescribed febuxostat (a non-purine selective inhibitor of xanthine oxidase) instead of allopurinol when his acute gouty flare settles. Studies indicate that the drug does not influence plasma protein binding of warfarin. The drug does not appear to cause any clinically significant interactions with warfarin or colchicine. Fenofibrate may also be commenced in this patient to treat both hyperlipidaemia and to help to lower serum uric acid levels.

CASE 75

Answers

1 Dactylitis, 'sausage digits', affecting the left little finger and right thumb, index and little fingers.

2 Dactylitis is most commonly seen in the context of a spondyloarthropathy, as was the case with this patient who has psoriatic arthritis. It is also seen in sarcoidosis, sickle cell anaemia and rarely, TB and leprosy.

CASE 76

A 23-year-old Caucasian woman went to her primary care physician complaining of swelling of the small joints of her hand and some aching in her feet. This was associated with early morning stiffness lasting over an hour. In addition, she had been troubled by increasing fatigue for the past 2 months that was not explained by any increase in her secretarial workload. She complained that her hands had felt cold during the past few winters but she did not describe any classical triphasic colour change.

In her family history she mentioned that her mother had had a long history of rheumatoid arthritis (RA) and she had a first cousin with insulin-dependent diabetes. There was nothing else of relevance.

On examination her pulse was 90 bpm, BP 120/80 mmHg and her heart sounds were normal. Examination of the chest, abdomen and CNS were unremarkable but examination of the locomotor system revealed slight, but definite swelling of the proximal interphalangeal joints and the metacarpophalangeal joints and some tenderness of the metatarsophalangeal joints. Just before concluding the examination the patient mentioned she had had some problems with her mouth (76).

Blood tests are shown in *Table 76*. Renal and liver function were normal.

QUESTIONS

1 What is the lesion shown in the image?
2 Does the positive rheumatoid factor clinch the diagnosis of RA?
3 Does the early morning stiffness in excess of an hour confirm the likely presence of degenerative arthritis?
4 In the absence of anti-dsDNA antibodies is systemic lupus erythematosus (SLE) unlikely?

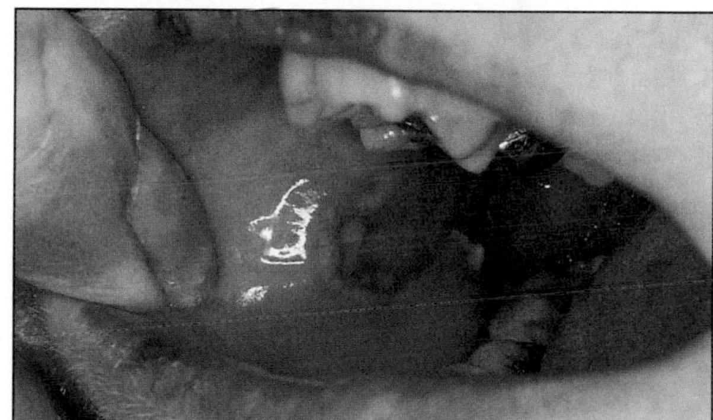

76

Table 76 Blood test results

Hb	11.2 g/dl	RF	1:160
WBC	5.6 x 10^9/l	ANA	1:1280 speckled
Lymphocytes	0.9 x 10^9/l	DNA antibodies	Negative
Plt	253 x 10^9/l	ENA	Ro and La positive

CASE 77

A 43-year-old man presented with swelling in the left elbow (77). He had no pain.

QUESTIONS

1 What is the diagnosis?
2 Discuss the differential diagnosis.
3 How should the patient be managed?

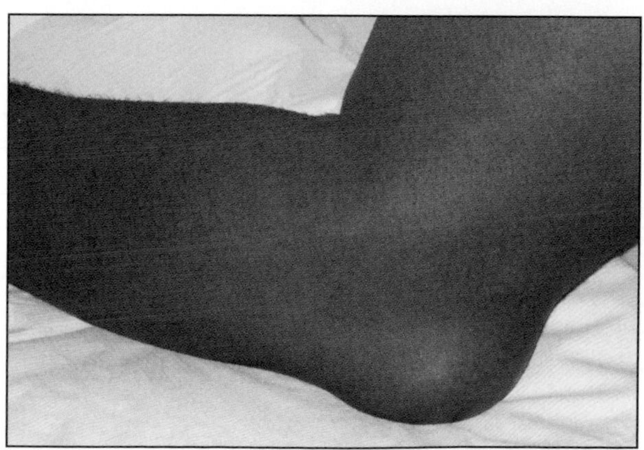

77

CASE 76

Answers

1 The figure shows a typical lupus mouth ulcer.
2 IgM rheumatoid factor is present in 70% of patients with RA but also in 20% of patients with SLE. An anti-CCP antibodies test may be useful here.
3 In approximate terms early morning stiffness of more than 1 hour is associated with synovitis; if less than an hour, with degenerative disease.
4 Approximately 30–40% of patients with SLE do not have anti-dsDNA antibodies. Provided the patient meets four of the 11 criteria proposed by the American College of Rheumatology, lupus may be diagnosed. These criteria do not have to present simultaneously.

CASE 77

Answers

1 Olecranon bursitis.
2 In this case the cause was mechanical. He used his elbows to smash tiles as part of a martial art. Although swollen, the bursa does not look acutely inflamed as you would expect in the other differential diagnoses – sepsis, gout and pseudogout. Olecranon bursitis can also be a manifestation of rheumatoid arthritis.
3 If there is any doubt about the possibility of sepsis, the bursa should be aspirated, and the aspirate sent for urgent microscopy, which should include analysis for crystals and a Gram stain with subsequent culture. In this case, however, there was no evidence of sepsis. Most traumatic olecranon bursitis settles with conservative measures – rest, NSAIDs and elbow pads. In this case, clearly changing his hobbies would help! In gout/pseudogout/inflammatory arthritis, injection with corticosteroid can be considered.

CASE 78

A 24-year-old female student presented to the local emergency department with flitting joint aches and a low grade fever a week after returning from Thailand where she had been on holiday. Her right wrist was particularly painful and tender along the palmar surface. She noted a skin rash on her forearm (**78a, 78b**) but could not recall being bitten by any insects. Examination of her chest, abdomen and cardiovascular system revealed no abnormalities. She had intended to visit her primary care physician to request pessaries for a vaginal discharge A speculum examination revealed a thick, mucopurulent, malodorous cervical discharge.

Questions

1 What is the most likely diagnosis?
2 What further investigations are indicated?

78a

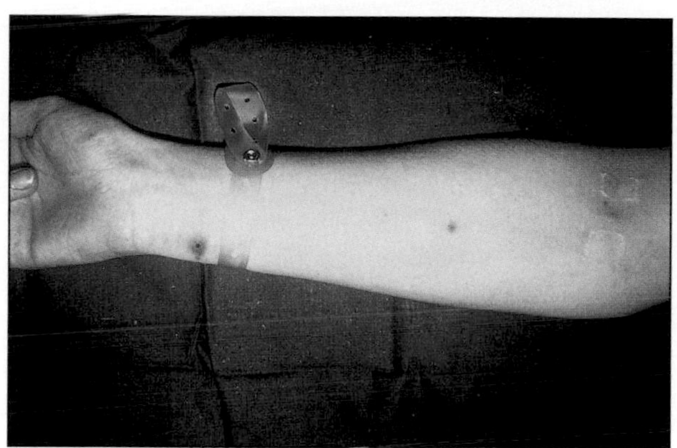

78b

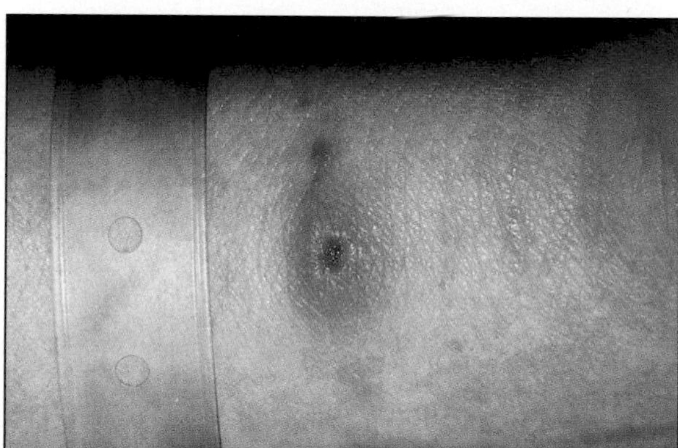

CASE 79

A 50-year-old man presented with a 6-week history of increasing pain and swelling in the Achilles tendon. He had just come back from a beach holiday where he played a lot of volley ball. He was fit. On examination there was a tender fusiform swelling 3 cm proximal to the insertion of the Achilles tendon into the posterior calcaneum. He could stand on his toes but it hurt to do so.

Questions

1 What is the cause of the patient's pain and what is a possible complication?
2 What is the differential diagnosis of posterior ankle pain?
3 How would you treat the patient?

CASE 78

Answers

1 Disseminated gonococcal infection is indicated. This patient presents with the classic triad of dermatitis, migratory polyarthralgia and tenosynovitis.

2 Further investigations would include: culture of mucosal surfaces (cervical cultures may reveal the diagnosis in this patient but rectal or pharyngeal cultures may be indicated if there is no obvious discharge), blood cultures, culture of first void urine and tests for other sexually transmitted diseases including chlamydia, HIV and syphilis. A pregnancy test is recommended as this may influence choice of antibiotic treatment. Contact tracing should be done.

CASE 79

Answers

1 The appearances are those of a tendonosis of the Achilles tendon and this site is typical. The likely cause is that he went from wearing normal heeled shoes to running and jumping in the sand allowing overstretching of his tendon. It can occur at any age but is more common in middle age. Ultrasound demonstrates the swelling and breaking up of the usually tidy alignment of the collagen along the length of the tendon. The risk is that it might progress to a complete tear of the Achilles tendon. This causes a palpable gap in the tendon. The patient is unable to stand on their toes.

2 Posterior ankle pain may arise from the insertion of the Achilles tendon. The pain is much lower. This may be a complication of a seronegative spondyloarthropathy. Pre-Achilles bursitis produces pain and swelling in front of the tendon. Acute pain higher in the calf may be due to a tear of the popliteus or gastrocnemius and is often brought on by sudden sprinting.

3 The patient needs to avoid walking without shoes and should have a heel raise. He should not run. Oral or local NSAIDs might help. Once the swelling has settled he can begin gentle stretching exercises. A local corticosteroid injection is absolutely contraindicated as it may increase the risk of a tear. In an active sportsperson the tendon is sometimes managed by surgical debridement of the internal structures of the tendon where the splits have occurred. If the tendon tears it is usual to place the ankle in a lightweight cast for about 6 weeks in slight plantar flexion. The patient should not weight bear initially. Corticosteroid injections can be used cautiously in enthesitis (alongside the insertion) or bursitis.

Outcome

The patient rested with a heel raise when walking and found oral NSAIDs helpful initially. He had local therapeutic ultrasound (although there is no convincing evidence that it helps) and then went on to gentle stretching and strengthening. He made a good recovery.

CASE 80

A 68-year-old man presented with hypertension with mild renal impairment and a 12-month history of suspected gout based on a history of transient left knee pain and mild swelling with a uric acid level of 380 mg/dl. He had an allergic reaction to allopurinol and then refused to be treated with any other uricosuric agents. Eight months ago he had a flare of knee pain and swelling and was started on colchicine 500 μg bd by his primary care physician. He missed two follow-up appointments as he went on holiday to the Caribbean. While there he continued to take colchicine once or twice daily but had episodes of painful swelling of the ankles lasting 3 weeks. Over the past 3 months he noticed general malaise, night sweats and progressive painless weakness of the legs and arms. On examination he has grade 4/5 power proximally in the upper and lower limbs.

The junior doctor is concerned that colchicine myopathy may be the explanation for his muscle weakness and general malaise. Preliminary results show a CK of 46 IU/l, Hb 10.6 g/dl, WBC 4.7×10^9/l, platelets 467×10^9/l, serum calcium 2.84 mmol/l, normal phosphate, CRP 33 mg/l, urea 9.0 mmol/l and creatinine 136 μmol/l.

QUESTIONS

1 Is this likely to be a colchicine myopathy?
2 What factors would increase the likelihood of colchicine myopathy in this patient?
3 How would colchicine myopathy be treated?

CASE 81

A 43-year-old chef from the Philippines presented to the local dermatology department with a curious V-shaped rash over the back. A biopsy indicated that he had some form of vasculitis. His ANCA test was, however, negative and he was simply provided with local steroid creams to apply. At this time his CK was noted to be a little elevated and over the course of the next year the level rose to approximately 1,000 IU/l. He was then referred to the rheumatology department where a careful history confirmed that for the previous 2 months he had been finding it more difficult to undertake his tasks as a chef, especially with respect to lifting and moving rapidly about the busy kitchen in which he worked.

In his family history he said there were no relatives with any history of muscle weakness and no features suggestive of any other autoimmune rheumatic diseases.

Examination revealed grade 4 proximal weakness in his arms and 4+ in his legs. His FBC showed an ESR of 47 mm/h but was otherwise normal. His renal and liver function tests were normal but his CK was 2,300 IU/l. Other investigations included a myopathic EMG examination and a muscle biopsy, suggestive of a polymyositis with necrosis and phagocytosis, and many inflammatory cells were evident.

Over the next 10 years the patient was treated with combinations of prednisolone and various immunosuppressive drugs including azathioprine, cyclosporine, methotrexate and IV immunoglobulin. In spite of this aggressive treatment his disease remained active and after about 5 years he began to develop some curious lesions on his elbows (**81**).

QUESTIONS

1 Is the proximal muscle weakness of polymyositis more common in the arms or the legs?
2 Are the inflammatory changes seen on the muscle biopsy sufficient to distinguish between patients with myositis and patients with muscular dystrophy?
3 This patient's ANA was positive to a titre of 1:160 but had it been negative would that have been a concern with respect to the diagnosis that was made of inflammatory myositis?
4 What are the lesions seen on his elbows?
5 Are there data from any controlled clinical trials that any immunosuppressive drugs are of value in the treatment of myositis?

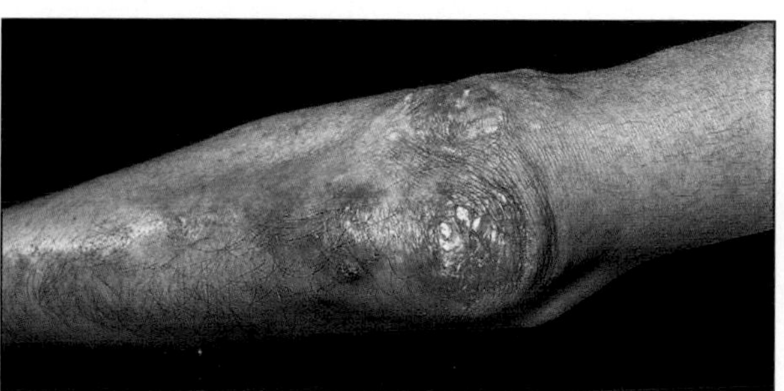
81

CASE 80

Answers

1 In colchicine myopathy, the serum CK level is usually greatly elevated (usually 10–20 times the upper limit of normal). There are only a few isolated reports of colchicine myopathy occurring in the absence of an elevated CK. The patient should be investigated for other causes of a proximal myopathy, particularly in light of his other abnormal blood results.

2 The presence of renal insufficiency.

3 Use the lowest possible effective dose or withdraw the drug completely. The weakness usually remits in 3–4 weeks after drug withdrawal.

Outcome

The patient was subsequently diagnosed as having sarcoidosis, which was confirmed by axillary node biopsy. His serum ACE was elevated. Ankle and knee aspirates did not reveal the presence of monosodium urate crystals.

CASE 81

Answers

1 The frequency of proximal muscle weakness in patients with inflammatory muscle disease is approximately equal in the arms and legs (in excess of 85% of patients).

2 Inflammatory changes indistinguishable from patients with inflammatory myositis can be seen in patients during the early phases of muscular dystrophy. The most useful distinguishing feature between these two conditions is the presence of muscle fibre hypertrophy, seen only in patients with muscular dystrophy.

3 Approximately 80% of patients with autoimmune myositis are ANA positive. The absence of an ANA should, therefore, give concern that inclusion body myositis, muscular dystrophy, or some other form of muscle disease could be responsible for the patient's weakness.

4 The lesions shown are due to calcinosis, which is rarely seen in adult patients with myositis. It is seen most typically in children with myositis and/ or adult patients who respond rather poorly to treatment and thus suffer long-term chronic disease.

5 There are very limited clinical trial data that azathioprine, methotrexate and IV immunoglobulin may be of use to patients with adult onset inflammatory muscle disease.

CASE 82

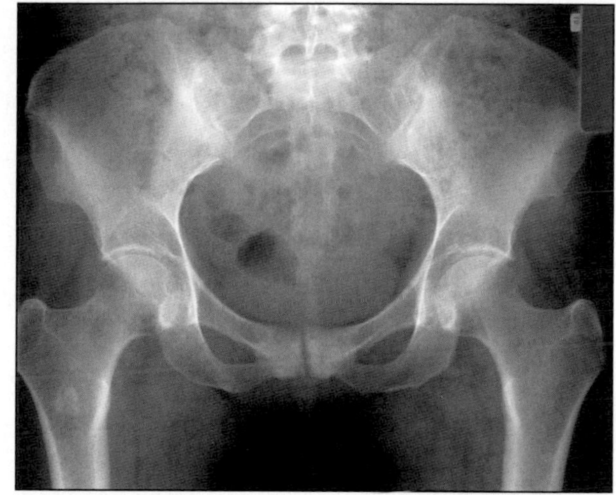

82

A 65-year-old woman was being investigated for persistent suprapubic pain. She denied other symptoms of urinary tract infection, and repeat urine cultures were sterile. She had a 20-year history of plaque psoriasis, but no other medical history of note. A pelvic x-ray was requested (**82**).

Questions

1 Describe and explain the abnormalities seen.
2 Discuss the options for management.

CASE 83

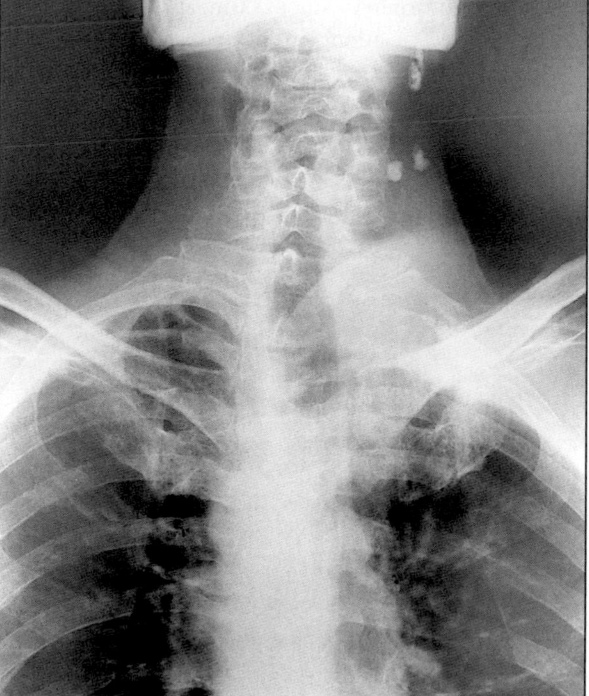

83

A 57-year-old female gardener presented to her primary care physician with a 4-month history of left shoulder pain but no limitation of movement. She was prescribed ibuprofen tablets. An ultrasound of the shoulder 3 weeks later was normal.

Over the ensuing 3 months, she noticed weight loss and anorexia. Her shoulder pain worsened and she noticed pain, and paraesthesia in the left fourth and fifth digits, the medial arm and forearm and weakness of the hand. Her chest x-ray is shown (83).

Questions

1 What is the most likely diagnosis?
2 What further imaging investigations are appropriate?

CASE 82

Answers

1 There is evidence of sacroiliitis, likely due to psoriasis. Patients may not recall pain if many years earlier. In addition, there are signs of psoriatic arthritis involving the pubic symphysis which is irregular, widened and has evidence of erosions. This was the cause of the pelvic pain.

2 This case requires active management of the psoriatic arthritis, with NSAIDs and the addition of adequate DMARD therapy.

Outcome

This patient was treated with methotrexate and sulphasalazine with resolution of pain after 2 months' treatment. This avoided the need for many invasive urogynaecological investigations.

CASE 83

Answers

1 A Pancoast tumour of the lung is indicated. These superior pulmonary sulcus tumours are usually squamous cell or adenocarcinomas.

2 Investigations to confirm the diagnosis and extent of metastatic spread include: CT scan of the chest and abdomen; MRI of the chest, which is superior to a CT scan in determining the extent of involvement of the brachial plexus, subclavian vessels, spinal canal and mediastinal nodes; fluoroscopically guided needle biopsy of the lesion; and fibreoptic bronchoscopy with sample retrieval for cytology. Sputum samples might not reveal cytological abnormalities because of the peripheral location of the lesion. In extremely rare cases (0.15–2%), active TB may coexist with a Pancoast tumour and confuse the diagnosis.

CASE 84

A 57-year-old man with severe seropositive rheumatoid arthritis presented to clinic during one such flare with a swollen, painful left elbow and tingling in the left fourth and fifth fingers. He had no fever or systemic upset.

He had failed therapy with methotrexate, sulphasalazine, leflunomide and etanercept. He required intermittent pulses of IV methylprednisolone to help control his joint pains. Nine months previously, a rituximab infusion had improved his joint pain and inflammatory markers for 6 months. Recent blood tests had shown sustained B cell depletion.

On examination, the left elbow was grossly swollen, but not erythematous. Flexion was restricted to 30°, pronation and supination to 40°. It was difficult to assess power at the elbow; however, he had good power for wrist flexion and extension, grip, abduction and adduction of the fingers. There was mild reduction of light touch sensation along the ulnar border of the left hand and the fifth finger.

The left elbow was injected with a mixture of 1 ml 1% lignocaine and 20 mg methylprednisolone. The patient reported no sensation of nerve penetration at needle insertion.

The x-ray of his left elbow is shown (84).

One week later, the pain and swelling had moderately improved; however, he noted progressive weakness and numbness of the left hand. At his 8-week follow-up appointment, he was noted to have marked weakness of the hand with clawing of the little and ring fingers and absent sensation over the ulnar border of the hand. The clawing had started 4 weeks after the steroid injection and had not improved. He denied any constitutional symptoms.

Questions

1 What complication has occurred?
2 What does the elbow x-ray show?
3 How should the patient be managed?

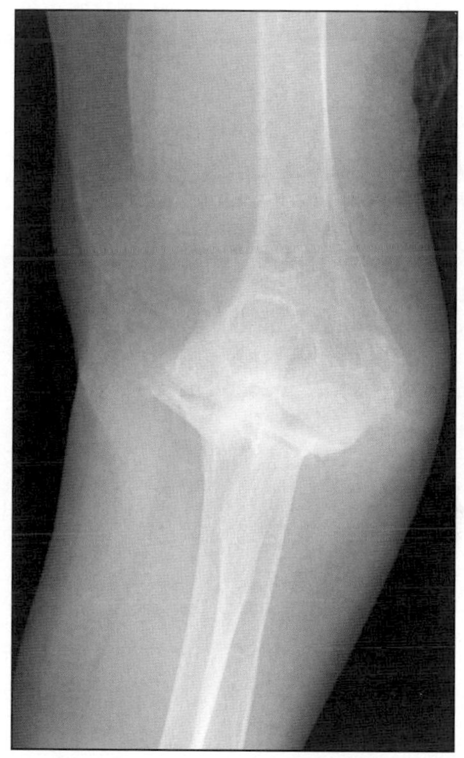

84

CASE 85

A 21-year-old man presented with a 2-month history of joint pain, particularly in his hands and feet, associated with morning stiffness lasting 2 hours. The ultrasound of the left second metacarpophalangeal joint is shown (85).

Questions

1 What does the ultrasound show?
2 What additional investigations should be requested?
3 How should the patient be managed?

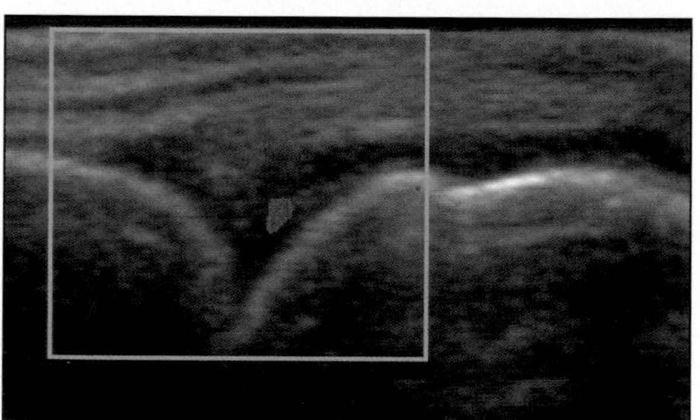

85

CASE 84

ANSWERS

1 The patient has developed an ulnar nerve palsy most likely secondary to compression at the elbow.
2 His elbow x-ray shows gross degenerative changes secondary to extensive erosive arthritis and marked obliteration of the joint spaces.
3 He should have nerve conduction studies, further imaging including an MRI and an urgent orthopaedic referral for consideration of ulnar nerve release and possible total elbow arthroplasty.

CASE 85

ANSWERS

1 There is synovial hypertrophy and hypoechogenicity suggesting an effusion, and positive Doppler signal. All indicate active synovitis. No erosions are seen on this image.
2 Further investigation would include x-rays of hands and feet to look for erosions, and chest x-ray. Blood tests should include inflammatory markers, FBC, renal and liver function, vitamin D, full autoimmune screen and viral screen.
3 The patient needs to start treatment with DMARDs. The choice of drug will vary depending upon immunology, but most rheumatologists would give an IM steroid injection, or short course of oral steroids, to get rapid relief of symptoms, and then introduce methotrexate, usually with another agent. In this case, the patient was rheumatoid factor and anti-CCP antibody positive and so aggressive treatment was started with methotrexate, hydroxychloroquine and sulphasalazine initially for 3 months, but because of inadequate disease control, a TNF inhibitor was added at that time.

CASE 86

A patient with classic features of early, active rheumatoid arthritis had hand radiographs (**86a**) and then an MRI (**86b**).

Questions

1 Is MRI usually more sensitive than x-ray in detecting erosions?
2 What is the clinical significance of these early erosions?

86a

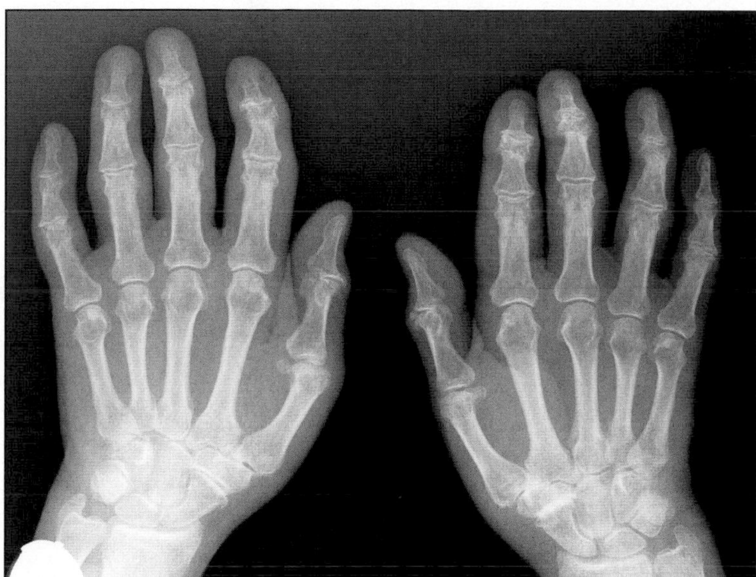

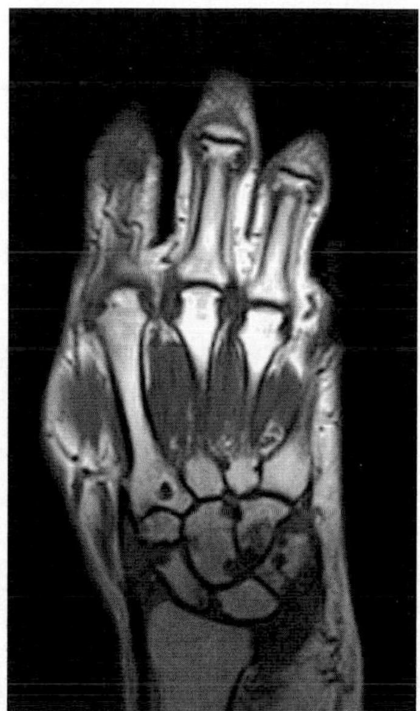
86b

CASE 87

A 51-year-old woman with long-standing dermatomyositis came for review to the clinic. For the preceding 3 months she had noticed gradually worsening abdominal tenderness. Examination revealed multiple small, hard, tender nodules over her abdominal wall. An abdominal x-ray was performed (87).

Questions

1 What does the x-ray show?
2 What is the diagnosis?
3 How should this be treated?

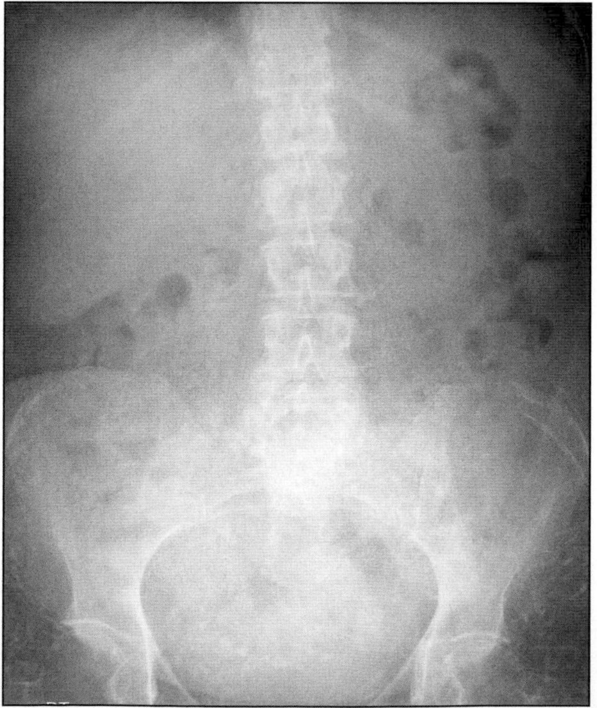
87

CASE 86

Answers

1 MRI is significantly more sensitive than x-ray in detecting early erosions. This is also true for ultrasound.

2 Although the clinical significance of early erosions remains uncertain, some data suggest the likelihood that they are reversible with aggressive treatment. This raises the possibility that they might be useful in guiding optimal therapy.

CASE 87

Answers

1 Multiple areas of calcium deposition.

2 Calcinosis cutis is indicated, which is a complication of dermatomyositis.

3 Cutaneous calcification as a complication of dermatomyositis is very difficult to treat, and there are no good trial data to guide therapy. It is more common in children. The main principle of treatment is to suppress ongoing inflammation, and there are cases supporting the use of methotrexate and azathioprine in combination. Calcium channel blockers and bisphosphonates have also been used.

87

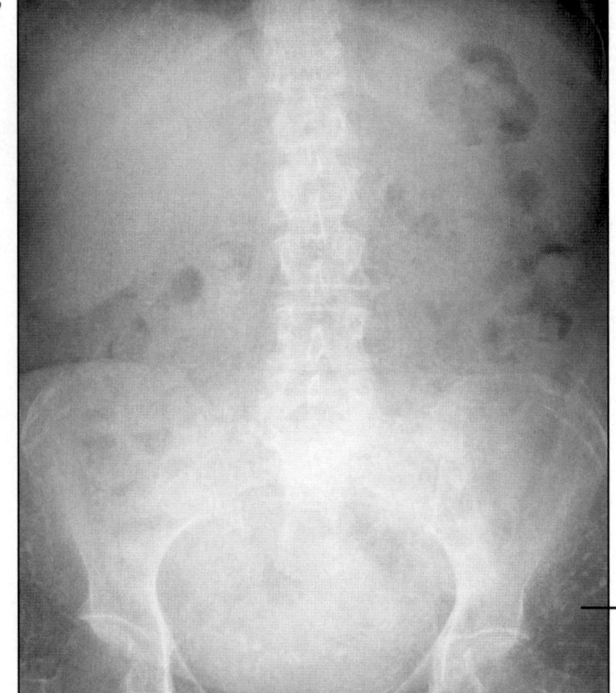

CASE 88

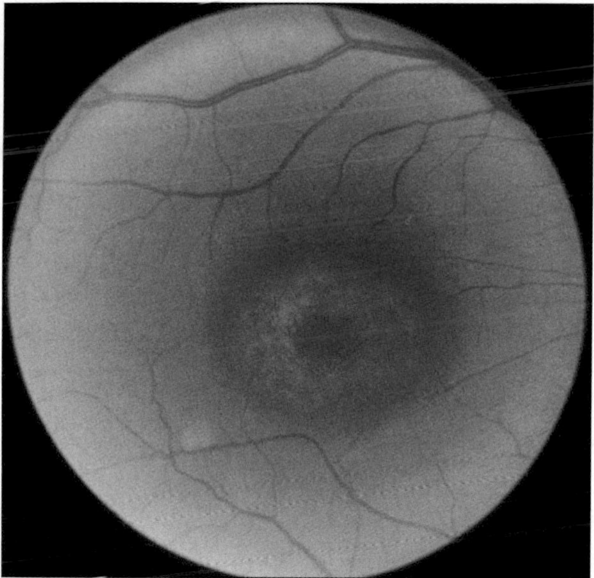
88

This female patient has SLE and had been taking hydroxychloroquine (HCQ) for arthralgia and fatigue for 4 years. She moved to the Gambia and was lost to follow-up for 6 years. While there, a local medical practitioner switched her to chloroquine which was more readily available.

In the year before she returned to the UK, she noticed progressive bilateral visual loss. Images of her retina were taken (88).

Questions

1 Identify the retinal changes.
2 What might have caused this?
3 How could this have been prevented?
4 What factors increase the likelihood of this condition developing?

CASE 89

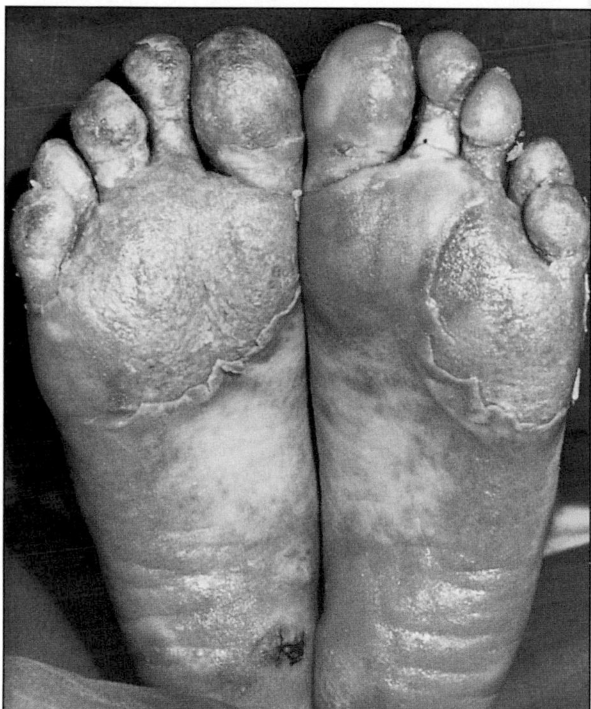
89

A 35-year-old bisexual man presented with a 4-week history of fatigue, malaise, painful elbows and knees followed a week later by the onset of a non-pruritic rash on the soles and palms. Four weeks before the onset of these symptoms, he had noticed burning on urination. He reported no other symptoms. His past medical history and family history were unremarkable. Clinical examination revealed a rash on his hands and feet (89). There were no nail changes or eye signs. His left elbow and right knee were mildly swollen with restricted movement. A sticky, mucus-like penile discharge was noted. The rest of the clinical examination was normal. Laboratory tests revealed raised ESR and CRP and positive *Chlamydia trachomatis* antibodies. Tests for HIV and syphilis were negative. RF and anti-CCP antibodies returned negative, HLA-B27 was positive. Knee and elbow aspiration each yielded less than 0.25 ml of pale-yellow synovial fluid which revealed no organism on Gram stain or routine cultures. Knee and elbow x-rays did not show any abnormal findings.

Questions

1 Describe the appearance of the patient's feet.
2 What is the likely diagnosis?
3 What are the important differential diagnoses?

CASE 88

Answers

1 Bull's eye maculopathy.

2 This was likely caused by the HCQ or chloroquine. These drugs bind to melanin in the retinal pigment epithelium causing cytotoxic effects.

3 Regular retinal and visual assessment including visual acuity, colour vision, central visual fields and slit lamp examination could have detected early signs of toxicity but visual loss might not be reversible even if the drug is promptly withdrawn. Policies for ophthalmological screening vary widely and take into consideration the relative risk of developing retinopathy including patient age and duration of therapy (refer to guidelines by the American Academy of Ophthalmology and the Royal College of Ophthalmologists).

4 The condition is more likely to occur with treatment with chloroquine. Risk factors for HCQ/ chloroquine maculopathy include maintenance doses of HCQ > 6.5 mg/kg/day or chloroquine > 3 mg/kg/day, treatment for over 10 years, liver disease and renal insufficiency.

CASE 89

Answers

1 The soles of his feet show erythematous, confluent, hyperkeratotic papules and diffuse yellowish hyperkeratotic plaques with desquamating edges such as seen in keratoderma blennorrhagicum.

2 Reactive arthritis (previously Reiter's syndrome) is the most likely diagnosis. This is a systemic disorder, originally defined as a triad of arthritis, urethritis and conjunctivitis and which usually follows an episode of either urethritis or dysentery. Only one-third of patients present with the classic triad of symptoms. Skin and mucosal involvement is observed in about 10% of cases.

3 The differential diagnosis of the articular manifestations includes other seronegative arthritides – ankylosing spondylitis, psoriatic arthritis, gonococcal arthritis and rheumatoid arthritis. Skin lesions may mimic pustular psoriasis and hyperkeratotic eczema of the palms and soles. The diagnosis may be confirmed by biopsy.

CASE 90

A 40-year-old personal assistant presented with lower back pain and intermittent sciatica down both legs. She gave a 25-year history of intermittent lumbosacral pain, particularly after running or standing for long periods of time. Examination revealed pain on lumbar extension, but normal neurological examination. X-ray of her lateral lumbar spine (**90a**) and lumbar spine MRI (**90b**) are shown.

Questions

1 What do the images show?
2 How should the patient be managed?

90a

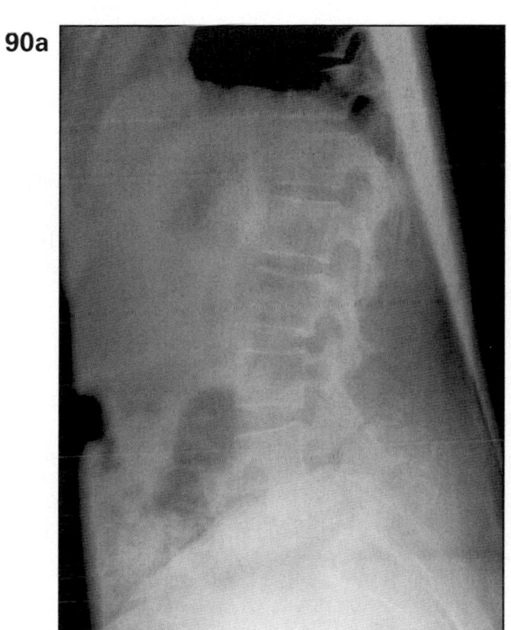

90b

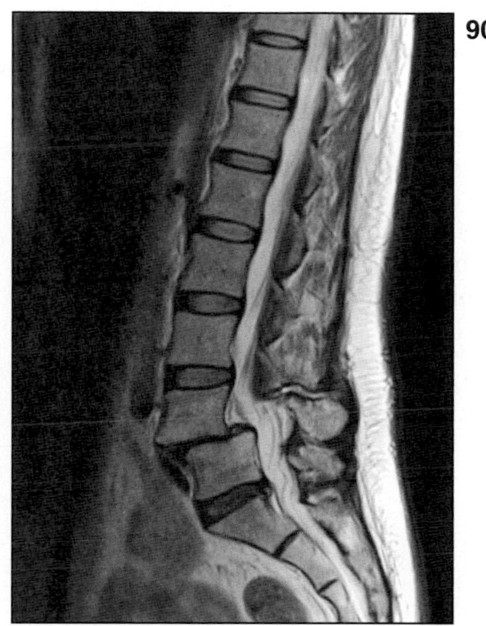

CASE 91

A 43-year-old hairdresser presented with a history of a shooting pain in the ball of her right foot whenever she walked. For the past 6 months she had been unable to work in her salon or wear stiletto heels because of the pain. There had been no preceding history of trauma to the foot, and no joint swelling.

Ibuprofen and paracetamol had not helped at all. On examination, mild pressure over the third web space caused significant discomfort. An x-ray of the foot showed no abnormality; however, an ultrasound revealed a Morton's neuroma in the third web space.

Questions

1 How does this condition arise?
2 What advice/treatment should the patient be given?

CASE 90

ANSWERS

1 The plain film shows a grade II spondylolisthesis at L4/5 with an identifiable pars defect. These findings are confirmed on the MRI, and in addition, there are degenerative changes in the L4/5 and L5/S1 discs. On this image, the central canal appears capacious.

2 Initial management should be conservative with physiotherapy and analgesia. Drugs such as amitriptyline and gabapentin may help with the neuropathic pain. Spinal injections can also be considered. Surgical fusion is reserved for patients who fail conservative management, but the associated degenerative discs make the need for this more likely.

CASE 91

ANSWERS

1 Morton's neuroma arises as a result of compressive neuropathy of the plantar digital nerve.

2 The patient should be given advice on appropriate footwear – broad, lace-up shoes, use of insoles such as a teardrop pad with the apex sited between the metatarsals to spread the metatarsals. An injection of corticosteroid may be of benefit in about 50% of patients. Definitive treatment involves surgical resection of the neuroma.

CASE 92

A 22-year-old female teacher presented to her primary care physician with a painful left arm. She had experienced mild and intermittent discomfort for nearly 12 months, but now the pain had intensified in the past 4 months and failed to improve with regular paracetamol and ibuprofen. She also complained of feeling moody and short-tempered. Her appetite had increased dramatically but she seemed unable to gain weight. In the last month she had noticed intermittent palpitations and a fine tremor of the hands.

Her primary care physician arranged an x-ray (**92**). The skin on her back had curious pale brown flat lesions which she had noticed since childhood. Her primary care physician identified these as 'café au lait' spots. Blood tests revealed a raised ESR of 46 mm/h, normal bone profile, liver function tests, urea, creatinine and electrolytes. Thyroid function tests returned abnormal with a low TSH of 0.98 mIU/l and raised free T4 of 28.2 pmol/l.

Questions

1 Describe the radiological abnormalities.
2 What is the unifying diagnosis?
3 How could the patient's bone pain be treated?

92

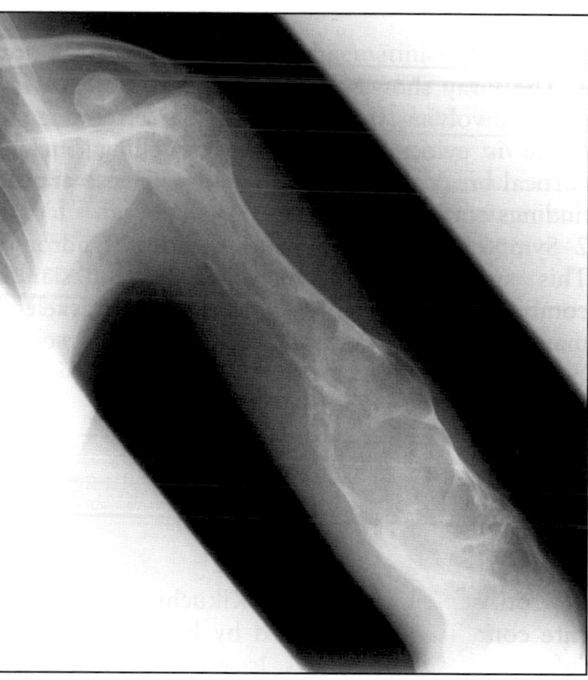

(Courtesy of Hussain *et al.* [2010] *Rapid Review of Radiology*, CRC Press.)

CASE 93

A 29-year-old Caucasian woman developed an evolving rash on her face and chest consisting of red, pruritic papules. Several months later she noticed swollen lymph nodes in her neck and began to develop fevers to 102°F (38.9°C) as well as night sweats and severe fatigue. A lymph node biopsy was performed, revealing necrotizing lymphadenitis.

The symptoms were responsive to courses of steroids but recurred when the treatment was tapered. Nine months after the first symptoms began, the patient suffered a grand mal seizure. On presentation to the university clinic, she was taking prednisone 30 mg/day and hydroxychloroquine 200 mg bd. There was active rash on her face, tender lymphadenopathy, a recent history of recurrent fevers, significant fatigue, night sweats, diffuse alopecia, Raynaud's phenomenon, oral ulcers and severe, disabling inflammatory arthritis to the point that she could not walk.

Laboratory studies were remarkable for leucopenia, a positive ANA at 1:1,080, low CH50 (15/50), and positive anti-Sm and anti-ribonucleoprotein by ouchterlony. Over the course of the next several months, methotrexate was initiated and increased to 15 mg/week. The major symptoms slowly resolved and the patient was able to return to work.

Question

Why was the lymph node biopsy performed, and what is the significance of the diagnosis?

and recent exposure to persons with TB as well

Appendix 1:

AUTOANTIBODIES

USE OF AUTOANTIBODY TESTING

Positive autoantibodies are neither sufficient nor necessary to make the diagnosis of an autoimmune rheumatic disease. For this reason, testing for autoantibodies should be confined to situations of clinical relevance and not used as part of a general screen. In the correct context, their detection can help with confirming a diagnosis and predicting prognosis. When used inappropriately, however, you are simply left with an abnormal blood test which can cause anxiety but on its own may well be meaningless.

METHODS OF DETECTION

Tests to detect autoantibodies usually involve immunofluorescence (such as the ANA [anti-nuclear antibody test]), or an ELISA (enzyme linked immunosorbent assay). ELISA allows for the quantification of an antibody (or antigen) of interest in a given solution. A fixed quantity of capturing antigen (or antibody) is coated on the surface of an ELISA plate. The test solution is added, and non-binding proteins washed away. An appropriate secondary antibody is then added which also binds specifically to the protein of interest. This secondary antibody is conjugated to an enzyme which can convert a clear substrate to a coloured product. This reaction can be quantified using a microplate absorbance reader, and recorded as optical density.

RHEUMATOID FACTOR

(See section on rheumatoid arthritis in Chapter 2.)

- Rheumatoid factors (RF) are antibodies which react with the Fc (constant) portion of immunoglobulin (IgG). All antibody isotypes can be seen, but most commonly, RF is IgM.
- Approximately 70% of patients with rheumatoid arthritis (RA) are positive for RF. Seropositivity is associated with more severe and erosive disease. On the whole, RF titre does not correlate with disease activity, although seroconversion to seronegativity after treatment may be predictive of good outcome.
- Positive RF is also seen in other conditions (see *Table A1.1*), and can be seen in the healthy population, with increased frequency in the elderly

Table A1.1 Conditions associated with a positive RF

Rheumatological	Infectious diseases	Other
Rheumatoid arthritis	Tuberculosis	Haematological malignancy
Sjögren's syndrome	Subacute bacterial endocarditis	Chronic liver disease
SLE	Leprosy	Chronic renal disease
	Syphilis	Old age
	Lyme disease	

ANTI-CCP ANTIBODY

- Anti-cyclic citrullinated antibody (anti-CCP) is another antibody marker of RA. It has approximately the same sensitivity as RF, but is more specific (90–95%). Anti-CCP appears particularly useful early in disease, where positive testing associated with a new onset of undifferentiated arthritis positively predicts the development of RA.
- As with RF, anti-CCP is associated with more aggressive, erosive RA.

ANTI-NUCLEAR ANTIBODIES

(See section on SLE and autoimmune rheumatic diseases in Chapter 2.)

- The detection of autoantibodies which react with components of the nucleus (ANA) is a hallmark of systemic lupus erythematosus (SLE), although positive ANA is also seen in a number of other conditions.
- ANAs are detected using immunofluorescence (**A1.1**) on Hep-2 cells. Results are reported as negative, or positive with a titre. Generally, a titre of 1:80 or lower is not considered clinically significant.
- ANAs bind to a variety of antigens, and different binding specificities result in different patterns (*Table A1.2*). Although these patterns are commonly still reported, the development of secondary tests to detect antibodies against the specific antigens has generally overtaken the interpretation of ANA patterns.
- In juvenile idiopathic arthritis (JIA), in particular oligoarticular JIA, the presence of ANA confers an increased risk of uveitis.

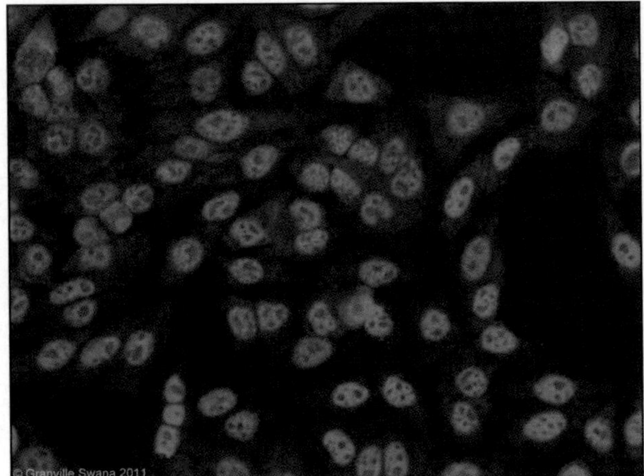

Fig. A1.1. Immunofluorescence demonstrating speckled ANA on Hep-2 cells.

Table A1.2 Common patterns of ANA staining

ANA pattern	Antigens	Disease association
Diffuse	Nucleosomes	SLE
Speckled (**A1.1**)	Extractable nuclear antigens: Ro, La	Sjögren's
	Jo-1	Myositis
	Topoisomerase-1	Systemic sclerosis
	Sm	SLE
	RNP	SLE
Nucleolar (**A1.2**)	Nucleolar RNA	SLE
Centromere (**A1.3**)	Centromeres	Systemic sclerosis
Rim or peripheral	DNA	SLE

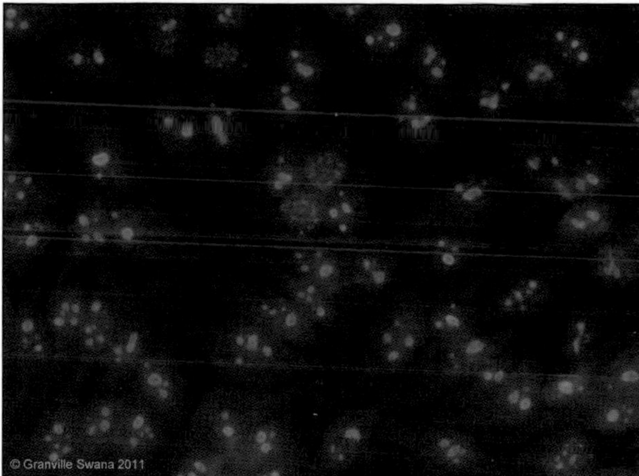

Fig. A1.2. Immunofluorescence demonstrating nucleolar ANA on Hep-2 cells.

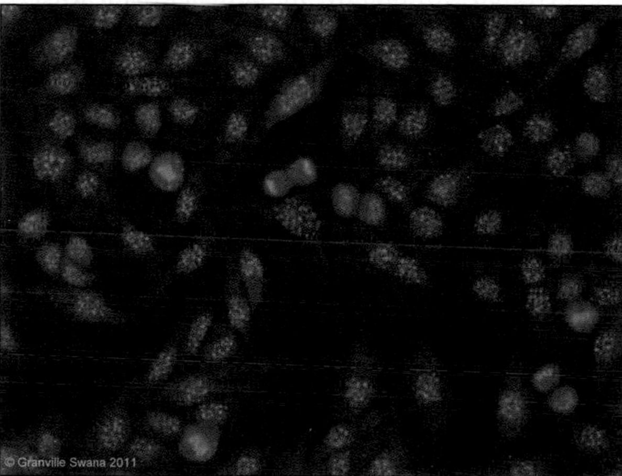

Fig. A1.3. Immunofluorescence demonstrating centromere ANA on Hep-2 cells.

ANTIBODIES TO SPECIFIC NUCLEAR ANTIGENS

The detection of antibodies to specific nuclear antigens is associated with more specific disease association (as shown in *Table A1.2*) and with particular disease manifestations. Occasionally, ELISAs detect antibodies to nuclear antigens in patients who are ANA negative by immunofluorescence. This is seen very rarely with anti-deoxyribonucleic acid (DNA) antibodies, but more commonly with some of the extractable nuclear antigens (ENAs) such as anti-Ro and anti-La.

Anti-dsDNA/anti-nucleosome antibodies

Anti-dsDNA antibodies are 95% specific for SLE, and their presence is associated with increased risk of renal disease. Unlike ANA, levels of anti-dsDNA antibodies vary with disease activity.

Anti-dsDNA antibody titre is most commonly measured by ELISA. In addition, the *Crithidia luciliae* immunofluorescence assay is also still widely in use. This test detects antibodies which bind to the dsDNA in the kinetoplast of the *Crithidia* (**A1.4**). It is relatively specific for anti-dsDNA antibodies. In particular, since the kinetoplast consists solely of dsDNA, anti-ssDNA antibodies do not bind.

Although the measurement of anti-dsDNA antibodies remains common in clinical practice, it is now generally accepted that antibodies to the DNA/histone complex, the nucleosome, are of more aetiopathogenic significance. Anti-nucleosome antibody assays also detect antibodies to histones and to combined histone and DNA epitopes.

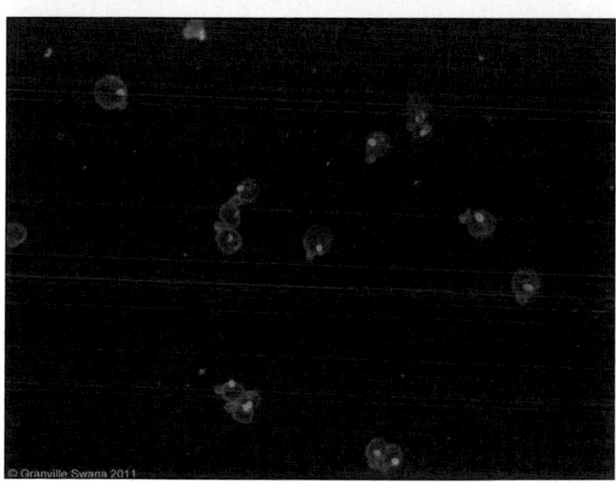

Fig. A1.4. Detection of anti-dsDNA antibodies on *Crithidia luciliae.*